70 Of The Barbecue Meat Recipes

That Will Allow You To Cook Up A Feast

Samantha Michaels

Table of Contents

Publishers Notes...5

ENJOY YOUR FREE DOWNLOADS?.....................................6

Introduction...7

Chapter 1 - Beef Recipes 8
Recipe 1 – Barbecue Bourbon Steak....................................8
Recipe 2 – Tomato Herb Marinated Flank Steak..................9
Recipe 3 – Grilled Steak with a Whiskey and Dijon Sauce..........10
Recipe 4 – Grilled Thai Style Beef Kebabs 11
Recipe 5 – Grilled Balsamic Steak.....................................12
Recipe 6 – Grilled Meatball Kebabs...................................14
Recipe 7 – Easy Grilled Veal Chops 15
Recipe 8 – Quick Grilled Beef Quesadillas.........................15
Recipe 9 – Spicy Lime Marinated Round Eye Steaks.....................16
Recipe 10 – Grilled Strip Steak with Garlic and Oregano 17
Recipe 11 – Grilled Beef Tenderloin with a Herb, Garlic &
Pepper Coating 18
Recipe 12 – Beef In Hoisin and Ginger Sauce....................19
Recipe 13 – Ranch Burgers 20
Recipe 14 – Three Herb Steak...21
Recipe 15 – Peppered Rib Eye Steak.................................22
Recipe 16 – Grilled Beef Tenderloin with Mediterranean Relish
....23
Recipe 17 – Jerk Beef with Plantain Kebabs......................24
Recipe 18 – Asian Barbecued Steak 25
Recipe 19 – Barbecued Chuck Roast..................................26
Recipe 20 – Barbecued Rib Eye Steak 27

Chapter 2 - Chicken Recipes 29
Recipe 1 – Rotisserie Chicken..29
Recipe 2 – Shish Taouk Grilled Chicken.............................30
Recipe 3 – Grilled Butter Chicken......................................31
Recipe 4 – Blackened Chicken..32
Recipe 5 – Grilled Herb Chicken Burgers...........................33
Recipe 6 – Grilled Chicken Wing with Sweet Red Chilli & Peach
Glaze 34
Recipe 7 – Grilled Chicken Koftas......................................35

Recipe 8 – Thai Grilled Chicken with a Chilli Dipping Sauce......36
Recipe 9 – Catalan Chicken Quarters..37
Recipe 10 – Thai Chicken Satay...38
Recipe 11 – Barbecue Chicken Breasts...40
Recipe 12 – Spicy Plum Chicken Thighs...41
Recipe 13 – Maple Barbecued Chicken...42
Recipe 14 – Spatchcock Barbecue Chicken......................................43
Recipe 15 – Chicken Tikka Skewers..44
Recipe 16 – Sweet & Spicy Wings with Summer Coleslaw..........46
Recipe 17 – Sticky Chicken Drumsticks..47
Recipe 18 – Jerk Chicken Kebabs and Mango Salsa......................48
Recipe 19 – Chicken & Chorizo Kebabs with Chimichurri..........49
Recipe 20 – Barbecued Chicken Burgers..50

Chapter 3 - Pork Recipes.. **52**
Recipe 1 – Pork Kebabs And Mushrooms...52
Recipe 2 – Barbecued Pork Steaks..53
Recipe 3 – Barbecued Pork Kebabs...54
Recipe 4 – Honey Mustard Pork Chops..55
Recipe 5 – Simple Grilled Pork Chops..56
Recipe 6 – Basic Barbecued Pork Spare Ribs.................................57
Recipe 7 – Southern Pulled Pork...58
Recipe 8 – Grilled Pork Tenderloin Satay.......................................59
Recipe 9 – Easy Teriyaki Kebabs..60
Recipe 10 – Baby Back Barbecued Ribs...61
Recipe 11 – Maple Garlic Pork Tenderloin.....................................62
Recipe 12 – Maple Glazed Ribs...63
Recipe 13 –Smoked Pork Spare Ribs..64
Recipe 14 – Bourbon Pork Ribs...66
Recipe 15 - Margarita Glazed Pork Chops......................................67

Chapter 4 - Lamb Recipes.. **69**
Recipe 1 – Lamb Chops with Curry, Apple and Raisin Sauce.....69
Recipe 2 – Grilled Lamb with Brown Sugar Glaze........................70
Recipe 3 – Mediterranean Lamb Burgers..71
Recipe 4 – Grilled Lamb Chops...73
Recipe 5 – Lamb Kofta Kebabs..74
Recipe 6 – Barbecued Asian Butterflied Leg of Lamb..................75
Recipe 7 – Summer Lamb Kebabs...76
Recipe 8 – Herb Marinated Lamb Chops...78
Recipe 9 – Grilled Indian Style Lamb Chops..................................79
Recipe 10 – Moroccan Leg of Lamb..80

Recipe 11 – South African Lamb and Apricot Sosaties (Kebabs) 81
Recipe 12 – Greek Lamb Chops...82
Recipe 13 – Grilled Rack of Lamb...83
Recipe 14 – Greek Burgers..84
Recipe 15 – Teriyaki Lamb Kebabs 87

Samantha Michaels

Publishers Notes

Disclaimer

This publication is intended to provide helpful and informative material. It is not intended to diagnose, treat, cure, or prevent any health problem or condition, nor is intended to replace the advice of a physician. No action should be taken solely on the contents of this book. Always consult your physician or qualified health-care professional on any matters regarding your health and before adopting any suggestions in this book or drawing inferences from it.

The author and publisher specifically disclaim all responsibility for any liability, loss or risk, personal or otherwise, which is incurred as a consequence, directly or indirectly, from the use or application of any contents of this book.

Any and all product names referenced within this book are the trademarks of their respective owners. None of these owners have sponsored, authorized, endorsed, or approved this book.

Always read all information provided by the manufacturers' product labels before using their products. The author and publisher are not responsible for claims made by manufacturers.

© 2013

Manufactured in the United States of America

ENJOY YOUR FREE DOWNLOADS?

PLEASE CLICK HERE TO GIVE ME SOME REVIEWS ON
THE BOOK ...APPRECIATE IT!!

MORE 70 BEST EVER RECIPES EBOOKS REVEALED AT
MY AUTHOR PAGE:-

CLICK HERE TO ACCESS THEM NOW

Introduction

Now summer is upon us most of us will be getting the barbecues out and using them once more. There are many benefits to be had from cooking food on a barbecue rather than in the kitchen.

When you cook food on a barbecue you find it tastes much nicer. The reason for this being that the intense heat produced by such equipment helps to actually caramelize the exterior of the food.

A barbecue not only helps to actually make the food look more appetizing by turning the food a golden brown color, but also you will find it helps to bring out more of the foods flavor. Of course if you would like your food to taste even more wonderful adding some wood chips to it can prove extremely useful.

You will often find that using a barbecue can prove more convenient but also easy to use. Once assembled you simply need to light the charcoal or turn on the gas supply and leave it for a little while to heat up.

Most people think that barbecues have only been designed for cooking all sorts of meat and fish on them. Yet there are plenty of models now available that allow you to cook a whole array of foods including vegetables as well.

Furthermore you will find that when it comes to barbecuing food you have a lot more cooking methods you can utilize. As well as cooking food by direct heat or indirect heat you can also cook your food using smoking and rotisserie methods as well.

Plus of course you will find that these types of equipment's enable you to cook meals for the family that are much healthier.

However rather than sticking with the usual sausage and burgers why not consider trying out some of the recipes that we offer in this book.

Chapter 1 - Beef Recipes

Recipe 1 – Barbecue Bourbon Steak

Although the flavor may be quite sweet, when teamed with a fresh crispy green salad you will find that this type of barbecued steak tastes wonderful.

Ingredients

4 x 200g Rump, Fillet or Sirloin Steaks
240ml Bourbon Whiskey
200g Dark Brown Sugar

Instructions

1. You need to lightly score the surface of each steak with the tip of a sharp knife on one side (diagonally). Then place into a shallow dish with the side you have scored facing upwards. Now you must pour the bourbon over the steaks and then over the top sprinkle on the dark brown sugar before then rubbing it in.

2. Once you have done the above you must now cover the steak up and place in the refrigerator and leave for 1 to 3 hours for the marinate to infuse into the meat. Around 15 minutes before you take the steaks out of the refrigerator you should get your barbecue going. Once the barbecue is hot enough and you have placed the grill about 6 inches above the heat you can place the steaks on to the grill sugar side down. Allow them to cook for around 4 to 5 minutes or until the sugar has caramelized.

3. Whilst the steak is going you should baste the side of the steak that is facing towards you with the remaining marinade before then turning it over. Just as with the previous side you should cook it again for around 4 to 5 minutes or cook until it is done to how you or your guests like it. Once the steak is ready serve immediately with a fresh green salad.

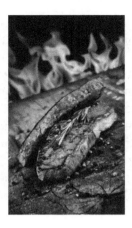

Recipe 2 – Tomato Herb Marinated Flank Steak

A very simple recipe that helps to make something that tastes truly amazing. If you can it is a good idea to allow the meat to remain in the marinade for at least 12 hours as this will help to make it much tender when it is cooked.

Ingredients

1 Medium Tomato
1 Shallot
60 ml Red Wine Vinegar
2 Tablespoons Fresh Chopped Marjoram
1 Tablespoon Fresh Chopped Rosemary
1 Teaspoon Salt
½ Teaspoon Freshly Ground Pepper
680 Grams Of Flank Steak

Instructions

1. In a blender put the tomato, shallot (which have both been chopped), the marjoram, rosemary, salt and pepper. Blend until they form a smooth paste and set aside covered in the refrigerator. If there is any of the puree remaining in the blender scrape it out into a sealable plastic bag into which you then put the steak. Make sure that you spend time moving the steak around in the bag so that it is all coated in the puree. Once all the steak has been coated you now place it in the bag into the refrigerator and leave it to

marinate for between 4 and 24 hours. The longer you leave the meat marinate in the puree the more flavor it will take on.

2. Once the allotted time has passed you should now get the barbecue heated up and set the grill above the heat at a height that it cooks the meat on a medium heat. Also make sure that you oil the rack first. Once the barbecue is heated up enough you should grill the steaks for between 4 to 5 minutes per side if you want yours medium rare or 6 to 7 minutes if you want yours to be medium. You should only turn the steaks one making sure that you brash the side that is already cooked with some of the sauce you reserved earlier.

3 As soon as the second side of the steak has been cooked you should turn it over again and brush it with more of the puree and then remove from the heat and place on a clean plate. Now allow it to rest for 5 minutes before then thinly cutting the steak crosswise. Before serving you should spoon on the rest of the puree.

Recipe 3 – Grilled Steak with a Whiskey and Dijon Sauce

Although this particular recipe contains alcohol when you cook it off you will find a lot of the whiskey taste has been removed instead a much sweeter oaky flavor is produced.

Ingredients

120ml Reduced Sodium Beef or Chicken Broth
3 Tablespoons Whiskey
3 Tablespoons Dijon Mustard
2 Tablespoons Light Brown Sugar
1 Large Shallot (Finely Chopped)
1 Teaspoon Worcestershire Sauce
1 Teaspoon Freshly Chopped Thyme
450 Gram Skirt Steak (Which has been trimmed and cut into 4 pieces)
½ Teaspoon Freshly Ground Pepper
¼ Teaspoon Salt

Instructions

1. Preheat your barbecue to a medium high heat. Whilst the barbecue is heating up you can prepare the sauce. To do this you need to combine in a saucepan the whiskey, mustard, brown sugar, shallot, thyme and Worcestershire sauce. Bring all these ingredients to the boil then reduce the heat so that a lively simmer is maintained.

2. It is important that you stir this sauce frequently to prevent it sticking to the sides of the saucepan and burning. Keep it simmering for around 6 to 10 minutes until it has been reduced down by about half. Then remove from the heat.

3. Now you need to cook the steaks on the barbecue. But before you do sprinkle both sides with the salt and pepper. If you want yours to be medium you should cook each steak for between 1.5 and 3 minutes on each side. However you should cook them for less time if you want yours to be medium rare. Once they have been cooked for the recommended about of time remove them from the grill and let them rest for 5 minutes before serving with the sauce.

Recipe 4 – Grilled Thai Style Beef Kebabs

The use of Middle Eastern seasoning in these kebabs makes them taste absolutely wonderful as well as helping them to become much more tender when cooked.

Ingredients

450 gram Beef Sirloin (cut into 1 inch pieces)
1 Bell Pepper (cut into 1 inch pieces)
1 Small Onion (cut into 1 inch pieces)

Marinade Ingredients

120ml Vegetable or Olive Oil
1 Tablespoon Rice Wine Vinegar
1 Tablespoon Roasted Sesame Seeds
2-3 Teaspoons Curry Powder
2 Teaspoons Soy Sauce
2 Teaspoons Sesame Oil

2 Gloves Minced Garlic
2 Teaspoons Dry Mustard
1 Teaspoon Hot Sauce
1 Teaspoon Cumin Powder
1 Teaspoon Sugar
½ Teaspoon Dried Ginger
½ Teaspoon Salt
½ Teaspoon Paprika
¼ Teaspoon Black Pepper

Instructions

1. Place the meat into a large sealable plastic bag and put to one side whilst you make the marinade. Best to place it in the refrigerator.

2. To make the marinade you combine all the ingredients above together in a bowl or jug. Once combined remove the meat from the refrigerator and pour the marinade directly into the bag and move the meat around to ensure that it is coated well. Replace the bag back in the refrigerator and leave it therefore for between 3 and 6 hours to allow the meat to become infused with the marinade.

3. When the allotted time has passed now remove the meat from the bag discarding it and the marinade. On to skewers you now place meat, onions and bell pepper alternately. If you are using wooden skewers then soak them in water for around 30 minutes, as this will prevent them from burning when placed on the barbecue.

4. To cook the kebabs place them on a grill over a medium to high heat and cook for 10 to 12 minutes, remembering to turn them occasionally. Once they are cooked remove from heat and serve.

Recipe 5 – Grilled Balsamic Steak

If you are at all conscious about the number of carbs you are consuming then you will find this recipe ideal.

Ingredients

Samantha Michaels

900gram Sirloin Steak (Should be about an inch thick)
240ml Water
120ml Soy Sauce
1 Small Onion (minced)
2 Tablespoons Worcestershire Sauce
2 Tablespoons Balsamic Vinegar
1 Tablespoon Dijon Mustard
2 Gloves Garlic (minced)
¼ Teaspoon Hot Sauce

Instructions

1. Please the steak either into a glass dish or a bag that is sealable. Now combine the rest of the ingredients above in a bowl or a jug and whisk thoroughly.

2. Once you have combined all the ingredients above together you then pour of the steak and leave to marinate for between 1 and 12 hours. When you are ready to cook the steak you should get your barbecue heated up and cook it over a medium to high heat.

4. When the barbecue is at the right temperature you should remove the steak from the marinade and place it on the grill cooking it on each side for between 5 and 7 minutes if you like it medium. Any leftover marinade should be discarded and once the steak is cooked to the way you or your guests like it you can now remove it from the heat and serve.

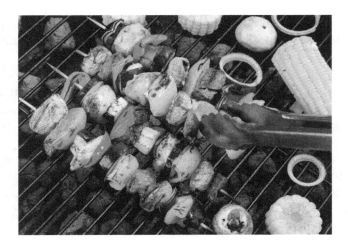

Recipe 6 – Grilled Meatball Kebabs

These meatball kebabs not only taste great when served on their own but also when you choose to put them into a sandwich.

Ingredients

450gram Ground Beef
1 Large Onion (cut into 1 inch pieces)
1 Large Red Or Yellow Bell Pepper (cut into 1 inch pieces)
115gram Dried Bread Crumbs
60ml Milk
75gram Parmesan Cheese (grated)
2 Gloves Garlic (Minced)
2 Tablespoons Dried Parsley
1 Tablespoon Dried Basil
½ Teaspoon Salt
½ Teaspoon Black Pepper
2 Eggs

Instructions

1. In a small bowl mix the bread crumbs and mil and let stand for 5 minutes. After five minutes squeeze the bread crumbs to help remove any excess milk and then combine this with the beef, cheese, herbs, garlic, salt, pepper and eggs and blend them together well.

After combining all these ingredients together you shape the meat into around 16 to 18 meatballs. They should measure around ½ inch.

2. Once you have created the meatballs you place them onto skewers one at the time and in between each one place a piece of onion and pepper.

3. Now you need to place the kebabs on to your grill that is lightly oiled to prevent them from sticking and cook them on a medium heat for around 10 minutes. Remember to rotate them every 2 to 3 minutes to ensure that they are cooked evenly. Once they have

been cooked properly you can remove them from the heat and serve.

Recipe 7 – Easy Grilled Veal Chops

This is one of the simplest and easiest barbecue beef recipes you may want to try. It tastes absolutely delicious especially if you serve it with some freshly grilled vegetables.

Ingredients

6 Veal Chops (Should be about 1 ½ inches thick)
3 Tablespoons Extra Virgin Olive Oil
2 Teaspoons Freshly Chopped Thyme
½ Teaspoon Salt
½ Teaspoon Black Pepper

Instructions

1. Preheat heat the barbecue and cook the veal chops on a medium to high heat. Whilst the barbecue is heating up you can now prepare the chops.

2. The first thing you need to do is coat the veal chops in the olive oil before then sprinkling over them (both sides) the thyme, salt and pepper. Once you have done this you now place them on the barbecue grill and cook on each side for between 7 and 8 minutes. Once they have been cooked for the allotted time remove from heat and serve.

Recipe 8 – Quick Grilled Beef Quesadillas

The great thing about this particular recipe is that it doesn't take that long to prepare so makes the perfect food to have mid week or as a starter for when organizing a big barbecue that lots of friends and family are going to be attending.

Ingredients

229gram Sliced Roast Beef
1 Can Black Beans (drained and rinsed)

689gram Monterey Jack Cheese
8-10 Flour Tortillas
172gram Salsa
57gram Freshly Chopped Cilantro
3 Tablespoons Lime Juice

Instructions

1. Turn on the barbecue so it is heated up to the right temperature for you to then cook these quesadillas properly.

2. Whilst the barbecue is heating up in a bowl combine the salsa, cilantro and lime juice and then set to one side. However before you do set it aside mix a third of this mixture with the beans in a separate bowl.

3. Now you are ready to start making the quesadillas. Onto one of the tortillas place some of the sliced roast beef and cheese before then topping off with a spoonful of the beans and salsa mix. Fold the tortilla over and place on the barbecue grill and cook for between 4 and 5 minutes turning them over once. Remove them from the heat as they turn golden brown and serve with the other salsa mix you made earlier.

Recipe 9 – Spicy Lime Marinated Round Eye Steaks

Another barbecued beef recipe that doesn't require a lot of preparation, but will still produce wonderful tasting food. Best served with grilled potatoes or a fresh green salad.

Ingredients

2 x 226gram Round Eye Steaks (measuring 1 inch thick)
Juice from 1 Lime
1 Teaspoon Garlic Powder
1 Teaspoon Cumin Powder
1 Teaspoon Ground Coriander
1 Teaspoon Salt
1 Teaspoon Freshly Ground Pepper

Instructions

1. In a bowl combine together the lime juice, garlic powder, cumin, coriander, salt and pepper.

2. Next trim of any fat that is visible from the steaks and place them in a plastic bag that can be resealed. But before closing the bag up pour in the mix you made earlier ensuring that the steaks have been coated well and leave in the refrigerator for 30 minutes.

3. Whilst the steaks are marinating you can start heating up the grill ready for cooking. Once the 30 minutes has passed you can remove the steaks from the bag and place them on the grill. Cook each side of the steak for 4 to 5 minutes before serving them.

Recipe 10 – Grilled Strip Steak with Garlic and Oregano

Another barbecued steak recipe that doesn't need a lot of preparation and so can be prepared and served to your guests very quickly.

Ingredients

4 Strip Steaks (1 Inch Thick)
3 Gloves Of Garlic Minced
1 ½ Tablespoons Olive Oil
1 Tablespoon Dried Crushed Oregano
¼ Teaspoon Salt
¼ Teaspoon Freshly Ground Pepper

Instructions

1. In a small bowl combine together the oil, garlic, oregano, salt and pepper then slather over the steak on both sides. Then place them in a dish that you cover and put in the refrigerator for 2 to 3 hours to allow the steak to become infused with the marinate.

2. It is important that when cooking these steaks you do so on the highest heat possible on the barbecue. Place them on the barbecue grill and cook each site for between 6 to 8 minutes. Once both sides have been cooked remove from heat and serve.

Recipe 11 – Grilled Beef Tenderloin with a Herb, Garlic & Pepper Coating

You may want to consider trying out this recipe first before you decide to serve to your guests. This will then help to ensure that you cook the meat properly.

Ingredients

2.26Kg Whole Beef Tenderloin
6 Tablespoons Olive Oil
8 Large Garlic Cloves Minced
2 Tablespoons Freshly Minced Rosemary
1 Tablespoon Dried Thyme Leaves
2 Tablespoons Coarsely Ground Black Pepper
1 Tablespoon Salt

Instructions

1. You need to prepare the beef first. This means trimming off any excess fat with a sharp knife before folding over the thinnest part of the meat so that it is about the same thickness as the rest. Of course if you want you could ask your butcher to do this for you. They will then tie it with butchers twine as well. It is also important that you snip the silver skin on the meat, as this will prevent it from bowing when it is cooking.

2. Once the meat is prepared now you need to mix the other ingredients together and then rub these all over the meat. Place the meat in the refrigerator whilst you prepare the barbecue to cook it on. If you are using a charcoal grill then build the fire on just one half of it. However if you are using a gas barbecue turn the burners up high for 10 minutes.

3. Before you place the meat on to the grill make sure that you coat it well with oil using a cloth that is soaked in oil between a pair of tongs. Once the grill has been coated with oil place the beef onto it and close the lid. After 5 minutes you now need to turn the meat over and repeat the same process.

4. After the meat has been seared (sealed) on both sides you now need to place it on to the side of the charcoal grill which is cooler or if using a gas barbecue turn off the heat directly underneath the meat. Cook for around 45 to 60 minutes or when a thermometer is inserted the internal temperature of the beef has reached 130 degrees Fahrenheit. Once it has cooked for the time stated now remove it from the heat and let it stand for 15 minutes (cover it over) before carving.

Recipe 12 – Beef In Hoisin and Ginger Sauce

Looking for something with a little kick, then look no further than this particular recipe. You can either serve this with some rice or noodles or some grilled Pak Choi.

Ingredients

900gram Flank Steak
240ml Hoisin Sauce
2 Tablespoons Fresh Lime Juice
1 Tablespoon Honey
1 Glove Garlic Minced
1 Teaspoon Salt
1 Teaspoon Freshly Peeled And Grated Ginger Root
1 Teaspoon Sesame Oil (Optional)
1 Teaspoon Chilli Garlic Sauce
½ Teaspoon Crushed Red Pepper Flakes
¼ Teaspoon Freshly Ground Black Pepper

For Decoration

1 Tablespoon Toasted Sesame Seeds
2 Chopped Green Onions

Instructions

1. At an angle thinly slice the steak across the grain so you are creating slices that measure around 1.25 inches thick.

2. Next in a bowl whisk together the hoisin sauce, lime juice, honey, garlic, salt, sesame oil, chilli garlic sauce, red pepper flakes

and pepper. Then pour into a plastic resealable bag and into this also put the steak and move it around so it is well coated by the marinade. Then place in the refrigerator for between 2 to 12 hours to allow the meat to become infused with the marinade.

3. When you want to cook the steak you should preheat your barbecue to a medium to high heat and thread the slices of meat on to skewers. If you are using wooden skewers soak them in water for around 30 minutes, as this will prevent them from burning when you place them on the grill. Any leftover marinade should then be discarded.

4. Cook the meat on the barbecue for between 2 and 3 minutes on each side depending on how you like your beef to be cooked. 2 minutes for rare to medium and 3 minutes for well done. Once the steak has been cooked sprinkle them with the toasted sesame seeds and chopped green onions before serving.

Recipe 13 – Ranch Burgers

This is a very quick and easy way to make burgers that not only taste wonderful but also look wonderful as well. Because very little preparation is involved you may want to consider getting your kids to help you make them.

Ingredients

900gram Lean Ground Beef
1 Pack of Ranch Dressing Mix
1 Egg (Lightly Beaten)
172gram Saltine Crackers (Crushed)
1 Onion (Chopped)

Instructions

1. In to a bowl place the ground beef, the dressing mix, the egg, crushed crackers and onion. Combine well together before then forming them into hamburger patties. You should be making the burgers as you allow the barbecue to heat up to a high temperature.

2. Once the burgers are ready and the barbecue has reached the desired you now place them on it. It is a good idea to coat the grill with some oil first to prevent the burgers stick to it. You should cook each side of the burger for 5 minutes and when done you serve them in a sesame topped bun.

Recipe 14 – Three Herb Steak

A very simple and quick recipe to prepare but the herbs used help to bring out even more of the steaks flavor. Ideal for serving to those who don't like their food a little hot.

Ingredients

2 Beef Top Loin Steaks (1 ½ Inch Thick)
2 Medium Red or Yellow Sweet Peppers (Seeds Removed And Cut Into ½ Inch Rings)
1 Tablespoon Olive Oil
Salt And Pepper To Season

Marinade

114gram Freshly Cut Parsley
60ml Olive Oil
57gram Freshly Cut Basil
1 Tablespoon Freshly Cut Oregano
1 to 2 Teaspoons Of Freshly Cracked Black Pepper
½ Teaspoon Salt

Instructions

1. In a bowl mix the olive oil, basil, parsley, oregano, cracked black pepper and salt to create the marinade.

2. Before rubbing the mixture made up over the steak (both sides) you need to trim off any fat. Once coated in the marinade you need to place them on a clean plate (covered) and put in the refrigerator for one hour.

3. Whilst the steak is in the refrigerator slice up the pepper before then coating with olive oil, salt and pepper. Put these to one side ready for when you start cooking.

4. As soon as you remove the steak from the refrigerator start up the barbecue. This will allow time for the meat to come up to room temperature making it much easier to cook. If you want your steaks to be medium rare cook for between 15 and 19 minutes (turning once during this time). However if you want your steaks to be medium then cook for between 18 and 23 minutes. Put the peppers on to grill around 10 minutes before you take the meat off. You should turn them once during this time to sure that they are cooked well.

5. After the time for cooking the steaks has passed remove from heat place on a clean plate sprinkle with rest of herb mixture before covering and leaving to stand for 10 minutes. To serve you simple slice the steak across the grain and then top off with some of the pepper rings.

Recipe 15 – Peppered Rib Eye Steak

Applying the dry rub mixture to the meat before cooking helps to make it taste more succulent. Plus it also helps to reduce the amount of calories and fat you are consuming.

Ingredients

4 x 285-340gram Rib Eye Steaks (Cut 1 Inch Thick)
1 Tablespoon Olive Oil
1 Tablespoon Paprika
1 Tablespoon Garlic Powder
2 Teaspoons Crushed Dried Thyme
2 Teaspoons Crushed Dried Oregano
1 ½ Teaspoons Lemon Pepper Seasoning
1 Teaspoon Salt
½ to 1 Teaspoon Freshly Ground Black Pepper
½ to 1 Teaspoon Cayenne Pepper

Instructions

1. Trim any excess fat from the steak then brush with the olive oil. Also snip the edges of the steak before coating to prevent them curling up when grilling on the barbecue.

2. In a bowl combine the other ingredients together before then sprinkling over the meat evenly before then rubbing it into the meat with your fingers. Place on a clean plate and cover the steaks once both sides have been coated in the dry mixture before then placing in a refrigerator for 1 hour.

3. To cook the steaks remove from refrigerator whilst the barbecue is heating up and when ready cook them directly over a medium heat and cook until they are done to the way you and your guests like to eat them. For steaks that are medium rare cook for between 11 and 15 minutes, turning them once. Whilst if you want yours cooked to medium then keep then on the grill for between 14 and 18 minutes. Again turning them over once during this time.

Recipe 16 – Grilled Beef Tenderloin with Mediterranean Relish

The Mediterranean Relish that you make to go with this particular barbecued beef dish really helps to create a more summery feel to the meal.

Ingredients

1.3to1.8Kg Center Cut Beef Tenderloin
2 Japanese Eggplants (Cut Lengthwise In Half)
2 Red Or Yellow Sweet Peppers (Seeded and Cut Lengthwise in Half)
1 Sweet Onion (Cut Into ½ Inch Slices)
2 Plum Tomatoes (Chopped)
2 Tablespoons Kalamata Olives (Pipped and Chopped)
2 Tablespoons Olive Oil
2 Teaspoons Crushed Dried Oregano
2 Teaspoons Cracked Black Pepper
1 ½ Teaspoons Freshly Shredded Lemon Peel
3 Cloves Garlic (Minced)
2 Tablespoons Freshly Snipped Basil
1 Tablespoon Balsamic Vinegar

¼ to ½ Teaspoon Salt
1/8 Teaspoon Ground Black Pepper

Instructions

1. In a small bowl combine together the cracked black pepper, lemon peel, oregano, and 2 of the minced garlic cloves. Once thoroughly combined together rub this all over the meat.

2. To cook the meat you need to place a drip tray in the bottom of the barbecue and around it place the hot charcoal. Once the temperature has reached the right level place the meat on the grill above the drip tray. As for the vegetables these should be placed around the meat directly over the coals, brushing them with olive oil first. Close the lid on the grill and allow it to remain closed for 10 to 12 minutes. By this time the vegetables should be tender and need to be removed from the grill.

3. Once the vegetables have been removed and placed on a clean plate and covered close the lid on the barbecue once more and allow the meat to continue cooking for between 25 and 30 minutes or until the internal temperature of the meat has reached 135 degrees Fahrenheit when a meat thermometer is inserted. If this temperature has been reached remove meat from barbecue place on a clean plate and cover leaving it to rest for 15 minutes before you slice it.

4. Now the vegetables have had sufficient time to cool down you can make the relish to go with the beef. Simply put all the vegetables into a bowl after coarsely chopping them and add to them the olives, basil, tomatoes, and garlic clove, vinegar, salt and ground black pepper.

Recipe 17 – Jerk Beef with Plantain Kebabs

You may think combining Plantain (a form of banana) with beef seems wrong, but the use of the Jamaican jerk seasoning helps to combat this.

Ingredients

340gram Boneless Sirloin Steak (Cut To 1 Inch Thick)
2 Tablespoons Red Wine Vinegar
1 Tablespoon Cooking Oil (Vegetable Is Best)
1 Tablespoon Jamaican Jerk Seasoning
2 Ripe Plantains (Peeled Then Cut Into 1 Inch Chunks)
1 Medium Sized Red Onion (Cut Into Wedges)

Instructions

1. Trim any excess fat from the meat before then cutting into 1 inch thick pieces then place to one side whilst you make the marinade for it.

2. Into a bowl place the vinegar, oil and jerk seasoning. Use a whisk to make sure that all the ingredients have been combined well together. Now divide the mixture into two separate amounts and use one half of the mixture to coat the steak. Then leave the steak to marinate in this mixture whilst you prepare the plantain and onion to make the skewers.

3. To make the kebabs you thread on to them meat, plantain and onion. Make sure you leave a gap of about ¼ inch between each item placed on the skewer. Then brush the onions and plantain with the other half of the marinade mixture.

4. In order to cook the kebabs you place them directly over the coals or turn the burners down to a medium heat and grill for between 12 and 15 minutes. It is important that you turn the kebabs occasionally to ensure that they are cooked evenly.

Recipe 18 – Asian Barbecued Steak

You may find the thought of combining fish sauce with beef a little off putting. However when combined with the other ingredients in this recipe it helps to make the meat much more flavorsome and tender.

Ingredients

907gram Flank Steak
60ml Chilli Sauce

60ml Fish Sauce
1 ½ Tablespoons Dark Sesame Oil
1 Tablespoon Freshly Grated Ginger Root
2 Gloves Garlic (Peeled And Crushed)

Instructions

1. In to a bowl pour the chilli sauce, fish sauce, sesame oil, grated ginger root and garlic and mix well together. Now set aside a few tablespoons of this mixture, as you will use it to baste the meat whilst it is on the barbecue.

2. Next you must score the meat and then place it in a shallow dish before then pouring over the remainder of the marinade you made earlier. Turn the meat over to ensure that it coated in the sauce completely. Then cover the meat and place in the refrigerator for no less than 3 hours.

3. To cook the steak you need to heat the barbecue up to a high temperature. Then just before placing the meat on to the barbecue brush the grill lightly with oil to prevent the meat from sticking to it. Now grill the meat for around 5 minutes on each side to have meat that is medium rare. Of course if you want your meat to be cooked to medium or well done levels then cook on each side for a little cooker. Whilst cooking brush over some more of the marinade you put to one side. When cooked let stand for a few minutes before then serving.

Recipe 19 – Barbecued Chuck Roast

Still hunkering after a roast dinner in the summer then this is a very quick and easy way of doing it. Plus doing it on the barbecue means much less mess for you to clear up in doors.

Ingredients

2.2 Kg Chuck Roast
240ml Barbecue Sauce
240ml Teriyaki Sauce
350ml Beer (Canned Or Bottled)
3 Teaspoons Minced Garlic

3 Teaspoons Freshly Thinly Sliced Ginger Root
1 Onion (Finely Chopped)
3 Teaspoons Coarsely Ground Black Pepper
2 Teaspoons Salt

Instructions

1. Into a large bowl mix together the barbecue sauce with the teriyaki sauce, beer, garlic, ginger, onion, coarsely ground black pepper and salt. Then place the roast into the marinade just made, cover and put into the refrigerator for 6 hours. It is important that turn the meat often whilst in the refrigerator to ensure that all of it is well coated.

2. You need to preheat your barbecue to allow you to cook the meat using the indirect heat method. Once the barbecue has had sufficient time to heat up now remove the meat from the marinade before then place on the barbecue grill on thread onto a spit. You should cook the meat for around 2 hours or until the temperature inside has reached 145 degrees Fahrenheit.

3. Whilst the meat is cooking taking the rest of the sauce, which you marinated the meat in originally and pour into a saucepan. Now heat it up until it starts to boil, and then cook for 5 minutes so it becomes reduced. You will then use this sauce for basting the meat whilst it is cooking. It is important that you baste the meat regularly during the last hour of cooking.

Once the time for cooking has elapsed remove from heat and allow to stand for 15 minutes before you then slice and serve. Remember to keep the meat covered whilst it is resting.

Recipe 20 – Barbecued Rib Eye Steak

Although the ingredients used to make this meal are quite sweet the fat in the meat and bacon helps to counteract it.

Ingredients

280gram Marbled Rib Eye Steak
2 Teaspoons Garlic Powder

1 Teaspoon Salt
1 Teaspoon Freshly Ground Black Pepper
700ml Cola Flavored Drink
950ml Barbecue Sauce
8 Slices Bacon

Instructions

1. Score the steaks on both sides using a sharp knife so that a diamond pattern is formed. Also make cuts into the fatty areas of the steak with the tip of the knife. Now sprinkle the steak with a small amount of the garlic powder, salt and pepper before then rubbing it into the scores you made previously. Do this to both sides of the steak.

2. Now place the steak into a shallow dish and pour over them the cola flavoured drink, cover and leave in the refrigerator to marinate for 4 hours. You should turn the steaks over every hour. Also during the last hour of marinating you should now cover the steak in a thin layer of the barbecue sauce.

3. After the steaks have marinated for 4 hours they are now ready to cook they should be cooked on the barbecue over a high heat. However before you place them on the grill make sure that it has been lightly oiled. Now cook on each side for about 4 minutes or until burnt.

4. Once this has been done either reduce the heat by turning the burners down or by moving the steak to a cooler part of the barbecue. Once you have moved the heat has been reduced place on top the bacon strips close the lid and then cook each side for 10 minutes. During the last few minutes of cooking again spread over a thin layer of barbecue sauce. Cooking until the sauce has become dried out and created a glazed effect to the meat.

Chapter 2 - Chicken Recipes

Recipe 1 – Rotisserie Chicken

A very quick and easy meal to prepare and then cook on the barbecue. You can either serve it as the main part of the meal or as a starter.

Ingredients

1.36 Kg Whole Chicken
57gram Butter (Melted)
1 Tablespoon Salt
1 Tablespoon Paprika
¼ Tablespoon Ground Black Pepper
Instructions

1. Season the inside of the chicken using a pinch of salt. Then spear it with the rotisserie skewer before then placing on your preheated barbecue. Make sure that the heat is as hot as possible and then allow the chicken to cook for 10 minutes.

2. Whilst the chicken is cooking in a bowl mix together the melted butter, salt, paprika and pepper. Once the mixture is ready and the 10 minutes have elapsed reduce the heat and baste the chicken with the mixture you have just prepared.

3. Once all the chicken has been basted you can close the lid and cook the chicken for 1 to 1 ½ hours. Whilst it is cooking don't forget to regularly baste it with the mixture as this will help to prevent the meat from drying out. You know when the meat is ready when the juices run clear after inserting a skewer into the thickest part of the chicken body or when you insert a meat thermometer the internal temperature of the chicken has reached 180 degrees Fahrenheit.

4. After the meat has cooked you now remove it from the barbecue and allow it to rest for 10 to 15 minutes before then carving it up and serving. Whilst it is resting make sure that you keep the meat covered up.

Recipe 2 – Shish Taouk Grilled Chicken

Bored with your chicken kebabs always tasting the same, then give this particular recipe a whirl.

Ingredients

907gram Chicken Breast (Cut Into 2 Inch Pieces)
2 Onions (Cut Into Large Chunks)
1 Large Green Bell Pepper (Cut Into Large Chunks And Seeds Removed)
60ml Fresh Lemon Juice
60ml Vegetable Oil
180ml Plain Yogurt
4 Cloves Garlic (Minced)
2 Teaspoons Tomato Paste
1 ½ Teaspoons Salt
1 Teaspoon Dried Oregano
¼ Teaspoon Ground Black Pepper
¼ Teaspoon Ground All Spice
¼ Teaspoon Ground Cinnamon
¼ Teaspoon Ground Cardamom
229gram Freshly Chopped Flat Leaf Parsley

Instructions

1. In a bowl whisk together the lemon juice, oil, yogurt, garlic, tomato paste, oregano, all spice, cinnamon, cardamom, oregano, pepper and salt. Then add the chicken and toss it through the mixture to make sure that all pieces are well coated. Then transfer to a large plastic bag (resealable kind is best) and place in the refrigerator for 4 hours.

2. Whilst you are threading the chicken, onions and bell pepper on to skewers start up the barbecue so it has reached the required temperature to cook these chicken kebabs. It is important that you cook the chicken over a medium to high heat for 5 minutes on each side. The exterior of the meat should be golden in color, whilst when you make an insertion in to the meat it should look white inside. Once they have been cooked through properly remove

kebabs from heat then sprinkle over some of the flat leaf parsley before serving.

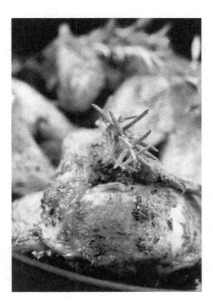

Recipe 3 – Grilled Butter Chicken

This particular recipe originally comes from India and is best made using a whole, which you or your butcher then cut up into pieces. The spices really help to make this dish much more flavorsome.

Ingredients

1.3 to 1.8 kg Whole Chicken (Cut Into Quarters And Skin Removed)
114gram of Pureed Onion
120ml Plain Yogurt
120ml Melted Butter or Clarified Butter (Ghee)
4 to 5 Cloves of Garlic (Minced)
1 Serrano Chilli (Seeds Removed And Minced)
2 ½ Tablespoons Ground Ginger
1 Tablespoon Ground Coriander Seeds
1 Tablespoon Oil
1 ½ Teaspoons Salt

Instructions

1. Combine together the onion, yogurt, garlic, chilli, ginger, coriander, oil and salt in a bowl. When combined together thoroughly now pour of the chicken pieces that have been placed in a shallow glass bowl. Now cover the chicken and allow it to marinate in the sauce for between 8 and 12 hours.

2. Next remove the chicken from the refrigerator and let it stand for 20 to 30 minutes. Whilst this is happening take half of the butter and melt it in saucepan and let it cook for 3 to 5 minutes.

3. Whilst the chicken is coming back up to room temperature turn on the barbecue so that you are able to then grill the meat on it at a medium to high heat. Make sure that the grill on which you place the meat has been lightly oiled first and then cook each piece of chicken for 25 to 30 minutes. You must make sure that you turn the chicken over regularly and baste it with the melted butter often. Once the chicken has cooked through remove from the grill. Now place on to a clean plate and pour over the rest of the butter.

Recipe 4 – Blackened Chicken

This particular recipe packs quite a punch. You will find that there is not only enough sauce for basting the chicken as it cooks but also to use as a dipping sauce as well.

Ingredients

4 Boneless And Skinless Chicken Breasts Halved
1 Tablespoon Paprika
4 Teaspoons Sugar (Divided)
1 ½ Teaspoons Salt
1 Teaspoon Garlic Powder
1 Teaspoon Dried Thyme
1 Teaspoon Lemon Pepper Seasoning
1 Teaspoon Cayenne Pepper
1 ½ Teaspoons Pepper (Divided)
320ml Mayonnaise
2 Tablespoons Water
2 Tablespoons Cider Vinegar

Instructions

1. In a small bowl place the paprika, 1 teaspoon sugar, 1 teaspoon salt, the garlic powder, lemon pepper, thyme, cayenne pepper, and ½ to 1 teaspoon of pepper. Mix well together then sprinkle over all sides of the chicken and set the meat to one side.

2. In another bowl you place the mayonnaise, water, vinegar and the rest of the sugar, salt and pepper. Once all ingredients have been combined together you put around 240ml of this to one side, which you place in the refrigerator to chill. The rest of the mixture is what you will be basting the chicken in.

3. To cook the chicken place over indirect medium heat on the barbecue. Remember to oil the grill first to ensure that the chicken doesn't stick to it then cook on each side for 4 to 6 minutes or until the juices that are released by the chicken as it cooks run clear. Don't forget as you are cooking the chicken on the grill to baste it regularly with the sauce made using the mayonnaise. After cooking serve with the sauce in the refrigerator.

Recipe 5 – Grilled Herb Chicken Burgers

As well as these burgers being low in fat they also taste extremely delicious. You will know if the burgers aren't cooked properly because they will be soft to the touch.

Ingredients

450gram Ground Chicken Breast
1 Small Carrot (Grated)
2 Green Onions (Minced)
2 Cloves Garlic (Minced)
1 Teaspoon Dried Parsley
1 Teaspoon Dried Basil
¼ Teaspoon Salt
¼ Teaspoon Freshly Ground Black Pepper

Instructions

1. Into a large mixing bowl put the ground chicken meat, the carrot, onions, garlic, herbs, salt and pepper. Mix thoroughly together. It is best if you use your hands to do this. Whilst you are mixing these

ingredients together then you should have the barbecue turned on or you should have lit the charcoal. So by the time the burgers are made you can then start cooking them.

2. After mixing the ingredients together you should make between 4 and 6 burgers from it. Before you cook them however place them on a sheet of wax paper and let them rest in the refrigerator for a few minutes.

3. Once the barbecue has heated up you must first lightly oil the grill before then placing the burgers on to it. To make sure that the chicken is cooked properly they should remain on the grill for between 12 and 15 minutes. It is important that during this time you turn them over at least once. You will know when they are cooked through, as the juices running out of them will run clear.

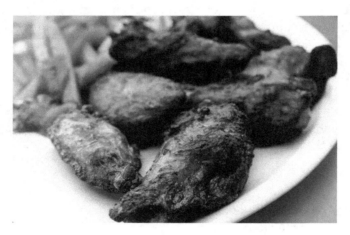

Recipe 6 – Grilled Chicken Wing with Sweet Red Chilli & Peach Glaze

The adding of the peaches into the marinade helps to counteract some of the heat from the chillis.

Ingredients

1.13Kg Chicken Wings
350ml Jar Of Peach Jam
240ml Thai Sweet Red Chilli Sauce
1 Teaspoon Fresh Lime Juice

1 Tablespoon Fresh Cilantro (Minced)

Instructions

1. In a bowl mix together the peach jam, the chilli sauce, the lime juice and cilantro. Take half of this mixture and pour into a bowl, as you will use this a dipping sauce to serve with the cooked chicken wings.

2. After your barbecue has reached the right temperature and you have sprayed the grill with oil to prevent the chicken wings from sticking place them on it. Grill the wings for between 20 and 25 minutes, remembering to turn them over frequently to ensure that they are cooked through evenly.

3. Only when the juices are running clear from the chickens can you then apply the remaining half of the sauce to glaze them. After applying the glaze make sure that you cook them for a further 3 to 5 minutes. Again you need to turn them over once during this time to make sure that they are well coated with the glaze.

Recipe 7 – Grilled Chicken Koftas

You can either eat these by themselves or you can use them as a filling for a sandwich or in pitta bread. If you are going to put them into pitta bread then warm the bread through first by placing it on the edge of the barbecue away from the direct heat source for a minute, turning them over after 30 seconds.

Ingredients

450gram Ground Chicken Breast
229gram Bread Crumbs
1 Egg (Lightly Beaten)
2 Cloves Garlic (Minced)
1 Tablespoon Cilantro (Finely Chopped)
1 Teaspoon Hot Sauce
1 Teaspoon Salt
¼ Teaspoon Freshly Ground Black Pepper

Instructions

1. In a large mixing bowl combine together the ground chicken breast, bread crumbs, egg, garlic, cilantro, hot sauce, salt and pepper. Then cover and allow to rest in the refrigerator as this will make it much easier to then form the Koftas (sausage shape patties), which you form around a metal skewer.

2. As soon as you have formed the Koftas around the skewer they are now ready to cook. Place them about 3 inches above the barbecue and allow them to cook for around 10 minutes. During this time make sure that you turn them frequently to ensure that they don't burn and that the meat cooks evenly. As soon as they are cooked you can then serve them.

Recipe 8 – Thai Grilled Chicken with a Chilli Dipping Sauce

You will find this recipe quite refreshing and with the dipping sauce it really adds a new element to the whole dish.

Ingredients

1.36Kg Chicken Breast (Cut Into Pieces)
120ml Coconut Milk
2 Tablespoons Fish Sauce
2 Tablespoons Garlic (Minced)
2 Tablespoons Fresh Chopped Cilantro
1 Teaspoon Ground Turmeric
1 Teaspoon Curry Powder
½ Teaspoon White Pepper

Dipping Sauce

6 Tablespoons Rice Vinegar
4 Tablespoons Water
4 Tablespoons Sugar
½ Teaspoon Minced Birds Eye Chilli
1 Teaspoon Garlic (Minced)
¼ Teaspoon Salt

Instructions

1. In a shallow dish mix the coconut milk, fish sauce, garlic, cilantro, turmeric, curry powder and white pepper. Then when thoroughly combined add the chicken pieces and turn them over in the sauce so that they are completely coated. Cover and place in the refrigerator for 4 hours or overnight to let the chicken pieces marinate in the sauce.

2. Whilst the chicken is marinating you can now make the sauce. To do this you place the vinegar, water, sugar, garlic, chilli and salt in to a saucepan and bring this mixture to the boil. Now lower the heat and let the mixture simmer for about 5 minutes. It is important you stir the sauce from time to time to prevent it sticking to the base of the saucepan and burning. Remove from heat and allow to cool before placing into a serving bowl.

3. When cooking the chicken on the barbecue make sure that the grill has been lightly oiled first. Cook each piece of chicken for 10 minutes on each side or until the juices start to running out of them clear. Brush them with a little of the sauce you made earlier before serving, whilst the rest remains in the serving dish and which people can then dip the chicken wings into if they wish.

Recipe 9 – Catalan Chicken Quarters

This is a Spanish inspired recipe where not only does the smoke help to enhance the flavor of the chicken so does the thick tomato sauce.

Ingredients

4 Chicken Leg Quarters
1 Onion (Chopped)
172gram Chorizo (Spicy Sausage Chopped)
1 Can Whole Tomatoes (Drained And Chopped)
120ml Red Wine
114gram Olives (Pitted And Chopped)
5 Cloves Of Garlic (Minced)
2 Tablespoons Olive Oil
1 Teaspoon Salt
½ Teaspoon Cumin
½ Teaspoon Cinnamon

¼ Teaspoon Cayenne Pepper
¼ Teaspoon Freshly Ground Black Pepper

Instructions

1. In a bowl combine together the salt, cumin, black pepper and cayenne pepper and rub over the surface of the chicken, making sure you get as much of this rub under the skin of the chicken as well.

2. Allow the chicken to rest in the refrigerator for a while (covered) whilst you start preparing the sauce to go with them. To make the sauce sauté the onions and garlic in the olive oil before adding the sausage, tomatoes and red wine. Allow this to simmer on a low heat whilst you are then cooking the chicken quarters on the barbecue. You should cook the chicken quarters until the juice runs clear from them, remembering to turn them over often to prevent the skin from burning.

3. Whilst the chicken is cooking you should now add the olives to the sauce and continue simmering it for a further 20 minutes.

4. To serve simply place one of the chicken quarters on to a plate and then pour over some of the sauce.

Recipe 10 – Thai Chicken Satay

Unfortunately this is a recipe you shouldn't be trying if you or someone you know is allergic to peanuts.

Ingredients

907gram Chicken Breasts Without The Skin (Cut Into Strips)
2 Tablespoons Vegetable Oil
2 Tablespoons Soy Sauce
2 Teaspoons Tamarind Paste
1 Stalk Lemon Grass (Chopped)
2 Cloves Garlic (Crushed)
1 Teaspoon Ground Cumin
1 Teaspoon Ground Coriander
1 Tablespoon Fresh Lime Juice

1 Teaspoon Muscovado Sugar
½ Teaspoon Chilli Powder

Sauce

2 Tablespoons Peanut Butter (Crunchy)
2 Tablespoons Peanuts (Chopped)
1 Can Coconut Milk
2 Teaspoon Red Thai Curry Paste
1 Tablespoon Fish Sauce
1 Teaspoon Tomato Paste
1 Tablespoon Brown Sugar

Instructions

1. You first need to make up the sauce in which the chicken pieces will be marinated. To do it get a large bowl and into place the vegetable oil, soy sauce, tamarind paste, lemon grass, garlic, cumin, coriander, lime juice, sugar and chilli powder. Make sure that you combine these ingredients well before adding the chicken and stir round until you know all the chicken pieces have been coated in the marinade. Cover the bowl and place in the refrigerator for one hour.

2. Whilst the chicken is marinating you can make the satay (peanut) sauce. To do this into a small saucepan put the peanut butter, peanuts, coconut milk, red Thai curry paste, fish sauce, tomato paste and sugar. Cook the ingredients on a medium to low heat, making sure that you stir it frequently and until it looks smooth. It is important that you keep the sauce warm after it has been made so turn the heat down as low as possible and cover.

3. To cook the chicken pieces you first need to thread them onto skewers and when this is turn place them on to the lightly oiled barbecue grill and allow them to cook on each side for around 3 to 5 minutes. Once the chicken is thoroughly cooked remove from the heat and either pour the satay sauce over them or provide it in a bowl which guests can then dip their chicken kebabs if they wish.

Recipe 11 – Barbecue Chicken Breasts

You will find that this particular recipe becomes one that you will use time and time again. When cooked correctly the exterior of the chicken becomes crispy whilst the interior remains moist.

Ingredients

4 x 250gram Skinless Chicken Breasts
Zest Of 1 Orange
1 Dried Chilli
1 ½ Teaspoons (Heaped) Smoked Paprika
1 ½ Teaspoons Dijon or English Mustard
3 Tablespoons Honey
3 Tablespoons Tomato Ketchup
1 Teaspoon Olive Oil
1/16 Teaspoon Sea Salt
Freshly Ground Black Pepper To Taste

Instructions

1. Into a bowl put the finely grated zest of the orange, along with the dried chilli (crumbled), the paprika, mustard, honey, tomato ketchup and the olive oil. Then after combining all these ingredients together add a pinch of salt along with some pepper then stir again.

2. Take out a couple of spoonfuls of the mixture made and put to one side. To the rest of the marinade in the bowl you add the chicken breasts. Turn them over so that they are completed coated by the marinade made and cover with plastic wrap before leaving to one side for 5 to 10 minutes.

3. Once the barbecue has heated up correctly you need to put the chicken on the grill but before you do make sure that you lightly oil it. When you place them on the grill make sure that the heat underneath isn't too high. If you notice the outer part of the chicken is starting to char quickly then move them over to a cooler part of the barbecue and reduce the heat if possible. You should be aiming to cook the chickens on each side for about 5 minutes, turning them every minute and basting them with some more of

the marinade left in the bowl. You should only remove them from the heat when they have turned a golden brown and are cooked all the way through.

The best way of testing to see that they are cooked all the way through is to push a skewer in to. If the juices that flow out are clear then you know the chicken is properly cooked. Remove from heat, then place on clean plates and spoon some of the sauce that you put aside earlier over them.

Recipe 12 – Spicy Plum Chicken Thighs

The plum sauce that coats the chicken thighs creates a slightly sweeter tasting barbecue sauce. It is important that you don't cook the thighs over too high a heat otherwise this could result in the sauce burning.

Ingredients

8 Chicken Thighs (Skin On And Bone In)
Salt and Freshly Ground Black Pepper

Plum Sauce

2 Tablespoons Peanut Oil
1 Small Coarsely Chopped Onion
4 Cloves Garlic (Coarsely Chopped)
1 Tablespoon Fresh Coarsely Chopped Ginger
1 Coarsely Chopped Thai Chilli
¼ Teaspoon Ground Cinnamon
¼ Teaspoon Ground Cloves
680gram Red or Purple Plums (Pitted and Coarsely Chopped)
60ml Honey
60ml Soy Sauce
2 Tablespoons Fresh Lime Juice
1 Tablespoon Granulated Sugar

Instructions

1. Before you do anything else you need to make the plum sauce. To do this in a medium size saucepan place the oil and heat it up. When it is hot enough add the onions and garlic and cook until they

are soft. Then add to these the ginger, cinnamon, Thai chilli and cloves and cook for 2 minutes. Now you need to add the rest of the ingredients listed above and cook until the plums have softened and the sauce has started to thicken. Then place the mixture into a food processor or blender and mix them until smooth. Pour into a bowl and allow to cool.

2. After making the sauce you need to heat the barbecue up to a medium low indirect heat for cooking the chicken thighs. Just before you place the chicken thighs on to the grill lightly oil it first and season the thighs with salt and pepper. Cook on either side until they turn a light golden brown between 1 and 5 minutes.

3. Now brush one side of the chicken with the plum sauce made earlier and turn the thighs over and continue cooking for 3 to 4 minutes. Once this time has elapsed brush the sides of the thighs facing you with more sauce and again turn them over to cook for another 3 to 4 minutes. You should continue turning and basting the thighs with the plum sauce until they are cooked through. You will find that they will be cooked through properly after 15 to 20 minutes. However if you are unsure just insert a skewer in to the thickest part of the thigh. If you notice the juices running out are clear then the chicken is cooked.

4. Please don't forget to keep the thighs at a good height above the heat to prevent them and the sauce from burning.

Recipe 13 – Maple Barbecued Chicken

You will find that the sweet flavor of the maple helps to really make this dish stand out and may have guests at your barbecue asking for seconds. To obtain the best results possible use a good quality syrup. Of course if you want to give this recipe a little kick then add some hot chilli sauce as well.

Ingredients

4 Skinless Chicken Thighs
3 Tablespoons Maple Syrup
3 Tablespoons Hot Chilli Sauce (Optional)
1 Tablespoon Cider Vinegar

Samantha Michaels

1 Tablespoon Canola Oil
2 Teaspoon Dijon Mustard
Salt
Freshly Ground Pepper

Instructions

1. Whilst the barbecue is heating up in a saucepan combine together the maple syrup, cider vinegar and mustard. Plus of course the hot chilli sauce if you are looking to give this recipe an extra kick. After mixing the ingredients together place saucepan on a medium heat and let the mixture simmer for 5 minutes.

2. Next you need to brush the chicken with the oil before then sprinkling on some salt and pepper to season. Then place them on to the grill and cook for between 10 and 15 minutes. As you cook them turn them regularly and each time that you turn them brush a generous amount of the sauce over them. Once cooked place on a clean plate and serve immediately. Any sauce left over can either be poured over the chicken thighs or placed a bowl, which the thighs can then be dipped into.

Recipe 14 – Spatchcock Barbecue Chicken

It is best if you get your butcher to cut the chicken up for doing this recipe.

Ingredients

1.3kg Spatchcock Chicken
3 Tablespoon Olive Oil
1 Teaspoon Paprika
1 Garlic Clove Crushed
Juice and Zest Of 1 Lemon
A Little Water or Beer to Taste
Salt
Freshly Ground Pepper
2 Lemons Quartered

Instructions

1. Whilst the barbecue is heating up in a bowl mix together the oil, garlic, paprika, lemon zest, salt and pepper. Once all these ingredients have been mixed together you brush it all over the skin of the chicken before then placing it covered in the fridge for 30 minutes to allow it to marinate.

2. When it comes to cooking the chicken on the barbecue you should cook it initially for 5 minutes on each side in the middle of the barbecue. Then move over to the side so that the heat cooking it is much gentler. It is important whilst the chicken is cooking that you turn it regularly and baste in between each turn with either beer or water. The best way of determining when the chicken is cooked through is to pierce between the thigh and breast bone with a sharp knife. When you do the flesh should feel firm and should look white.

You should be cooking each side of the chicken for between 20 and 30 minutes. Plus place something over the top, as the steam produced will help the chicken to cook through.

3. Once the chicken has cooked you now need to remove it from the heat and leave it to rest. Make sure that you cover it with foil and leave it to rest for around 10 to 15 minutes. Once this time has passed cut it up into pieces and drizzle some lemon juice, oil, salt, pepper and paprika over them. Then serve on a fresh plate with the lemon quarters.

Recipe 15 – Chicken Tikka Skewers

As well as being a quick and easy dish to prepare for your barbecue this summer, this particular recipe is also low in calories.

Ingredients

4 Skinless Boneless Chicken Breasts Cut Into Cubes
150gram Low Fat Natural Yogurt
2 Tablespoon Hot Curry Paste
250gram Cherry Tomatoes
4 Wholemeal Chapattis
½ Cucumber Cut In Half Lengthways, Deseeded and then Sliced
1 Red Onion Thinly Sliced

Handful Coriander Leaves Chopped
Juice 1 Lemon
50gram Lamb's Lettuce or Pea Shoots

Instructions

1. Place the wooden skewers (8 in all) in some water in a bowl to soak. After doing this you need to place the yogurt and curry paste in a bowl and mix together then to this you add the cubes of chicken. Make sure that you stir the chicken into the mixture well to ensure all pieces are coated. Now cover the top of the bowl and place in the refrigerator to marinate for an hour or so.

2. Next in another bowl place the cucumber, red onion, coriander and lemon and toss them altogether. Again place this bowl in the refrigerator (covered over) and leave there until you are ready to serve the chicken.

3. Whilst the barbecue is heated up now you need to start preparing the skewers. You must make sure that you shake off any excess marinade before then threading the pieces of chicken on to the skewers. After threading on a piece of chicken now thread on a cherry tomato and do this until all skewers have been used.

4. Once the Chicken Tikka skewers are ready and the barbecue has heated up you are now ready to start cooking. You should keep the skewers on the barbecue for between 15 and 20 minutes, making sure that you turn them regularly so that they get cooked through and become a nice brown color.

5. When it comes to serving the skewers place them to one side on a clean plate to rest for a few minutes whilst you prepare the salad. Into the salad before serving mix the lettuce and pea shoots and divide this equally between four plates and on top of which you then place two of the skewers. Serve them with chapattis that have been warmed through on the barbecue. The best way to warm the chapattis on the barbecue is to wrap them in some aluminum foil.

Recipe 16 – Sweet & Spicy Wings with Summer Coleslaw

Just like many other recipes in this book this is one that is very quick and easy to make and will certainly help to add a little spice to your barbecue this summer.

Ingredients

1kg Chicken Wings
4 Tablespoon Curry Paste (Tikka would be wonderful)
3 Tablespoon Mango Chutney
200g Sliced Radishes
1 Cucumber Halved Lengthways And Sliced
1 Small Bunch Roughly Chopped Mint
Juice Of 1 Lemon

Instructions

1. Start getting the barbecue heated up. Now in to a large bowl place the curry paste and 2 tablespoons of the mango chutney with a little salt and pepper to season, then stir well.

2. Place the chicken wings in the mixture and toss around so that they are all well coated and then leave to marinate for a short while.

3. Now place on to the barbecue griddle making sure that the surface has been lightly oiled first to prevent the chicken sticking to it. Now cook for between 40 and 45 minutes, turning occasionally until all sides are golden brown and the wings are cooked through. The quickest way to determine if the wings have been cooked through is to stick a skewer into the thickest part and when removed do the juices run clear.

4. Finally just before you are about to serve the chicken wings in another bowl place the radishes, cucumber, mint, the rest of the mango chutney and the lemon juice and stir thoroughly. Now place the chicken wings on a clean plate and then beside it place the freshly made coleslaw.

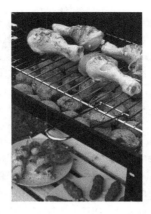

Recipe 17 – Sticky Chicken Drumsticks

This isn't only a recipe that kids will enjoy eating so will many adults, especially those with somewhat of a sweet tooth.

Ingredients

8 Chicken Drumsticks
2 Tablespoon Soy Sauce
1 Tablespoon Honey
1 Tablespoon Olive Oil
1 Tablespoon Tomato Puree
1 Tablespoon Dijon Mustard

Instructions

1. You need to make 3 slashes into each chicken drumstick as this will then help the meat to absorb quite a bit of the marinade you are about to make. Then place the drumsticks into a shallow dish.

2. To make the marinade you need to place the soy sauce, honey, olive oil, mustard and tomato puree into a bowl and whisk together thoroughly. Once all these ingredients have been combined pour some over the drumsticks before turning them over and pouring the remainder of the marinade over them. Once this has been done you must place them in the refrigerator overnight (remembering to cover them).

3. Whilst the barbecue is heating up ready for you to cook the drumsticks remove them from the refrigerator and allow them to come up to room temperature. When the barbecue is heated up sufficiently you can now place the drumsticks on to the grill. Although there is oil in the marinade don't forget to brush some over the grill to prevent the chicken drumsticks from sticking to them.

4. It is important that you cook these for around 35 minutes or until the juice inside them starts to run clear. Also it is important to remember to turn them over regularly to prevent the exterior from becoming burnt and also to ensure that they cook right through. Once they are cooked now place them on a clean plate and serve to your waiting guests.

Recipe 18 – Jerk Chicken Kebabs and Mango Salsa

The inclusion of a mango salsa with these kebabs helps to take some of the kick out of the spices used in making the Jerk Chicken.

Ingredients

Jerk Chicken
4 Skinless Chicken Breasts Cut Into Chunks
2 Teaspoon Jerk Seasoning
1 Tablespoon Olive Oil
Juice of 1 Lime
1 Large Yellow Pepper Cut Into 2cm Cubes

Mango Salsa

320g Mango Diced
1 Large Red Pepper Deseeded and Diced
Bunch Spring Onions Finely Chopped
1 Red Chilli Chopped (This Is Optional)

Instructions

1. In a bowl place the jerk seasoning, olive oil and lime juice and then mix thoroughly together. A whisk would be best to do this. Then once all these ingredients have been thoroughly combined

toss the chunks of chicken in it and place in the refrigerator for at least 20 minutes. However if you really want the meat to absorb as much of the marinade as possible then it is best to leave it in the refrigerator for at least 24 hours.

2. Once the meat has time to marinade you are now ready to start cooking it. But whilst the barbecue is heating up you can now start making the salsa. To do this you simply place all the ingredients mentioned above in a bowl and stir together. Add a little salt and pepper to season then place in the refrigerator until you are ready to serve it with the kebabs.

3. To make the kebabs you need some wooden skewers, which have been left in some water for at least 30 minutes. Remember doing this will prevent them from burning. Now on to each skewer you thread a piece of chicken followed by a piece of the yellow pepper. You should be aiming to put on each of the 8 skewers 3 pieces of meat and 3 pieces of pepper.

4. Once the kebabs have been made and the barbecue is hot enough you can start cooking them. Each side of the kebab should be cooked for around 8 minutes. This will not only ensure that they are cooked through but also helps to create a little charring on them. Once they are cooked place two kebabs on a plate and add some salsa

Recipe 19 – Chicken & Chorizo Kebabs with Chimichurri

This really is something different and the chorizo along with the Chimichurri helps to provide a little bit of spice to these kebabs.

Ingredients

250g Chicken Breast Cut Into Chunks
250g Chorizo Cut Into Chunks
Olive Oil For Brushing The Kebabs

Chimichurri

4 Tablespoon Freshly Chopped Parsley
1 Red Chilli Chopped

1 Garlic Clove Chopped
2 Teaspoon Dried Oregano
2 Teaspoon Smoked Paprika
5 Tablespoon Olive Oil
2 Tablespoon Red Wine Vinegar

Instructions

1. On to several skewers you need to place chunks of the chicken and chorizo sausage and then lightly season with some salt and pepper before then brushing with some olive oil before placing on to the barbecue. It is important that whilst cooking these for around 10 minutes you turn them regularly to prevent them from becoming burnt.

2. Whilst the kebabs are cooking you can now make the Chimichurri sauce. This is very simple to do simply place all the ingredients above in a bowl and then whisk thoroughly. By the time you have done this the kebabs should have cooked and will be ready to serve. Simply place two kebabs on each clean plate and serve a small bowl of the Chimichurri beside them.

Recipe 20 – Barbecued Chicken Burgers

If you are having a last minute barbecue one summer evening you will be able to serve these very quickly to your family and friends.

Ingredients

4 Skinless Chicken Breasts
4 Tablespoon Tomato Ketchup
4 Tablespoon Brown Sauce
2 Teaspoon Clear Honey
2 Garlic Cloves Crushed
Splash Of Chilli Sauce (Optional)

Instructions

1. In a large bowl combine together the tomato ketchup, brown sauce, honey and garlic cloves. It is at this time you also add the chilli sauce if you wish this will give this sweet recipe a little kick.

Once this has been done put take some of the mixture out as this you can then use as a sauce that people can put on to the chicken burgers after they have cooked.

2. Next you need to cut halfway into the thickest part of the chicken breast and then open it up in the same way you would a book. You should flatten the breasts down slightly using the palm of your hand then place them in the bowl with the marinade and toss to ensure all parts of the breast are coated with it. Now place in the refrigerator for around 20 minutes (remembering to cover the breasts over).

3. Whilst the barbecue is heating up you now need to remove the chicken from the refrigerator to bring it back up to room temperature. Once the barbecue is heated up sufficiently you can now place the chicken breasts on the grill, remembering to brush it lightly with oil first. You should cook each chicken breast for around 10 minutes or until they are cooked through. Also whilst cooking the breasts remember to turn them over regularly to help the marinade to become sticky and also to help prevent the meat from burning.

4. Once they are cooked you can place them in buns with slices of bacon (cooked) and some lettuce and slices of tomato and onion. Plus don't forget to add a dollop of the sauce you put to one side earlier.

Chapter 3 - Pork Recipes

Recipe 1 – Pork Kebabs And Mushrooms

You will find that not only do these kebabs take very little time to prepare but also take very little time to cook, but make a great addition to any barbecue.

Ingredients

450gram Pork Fillet Cut Into 1 Inch Chunks
4 Tablespoon Olive Oil
2 Garlic Cloves Crushed
24 Button Mushrooms
24 Fresh Sage Leaves
Salt
Freshly Ground Black Pepper

Instructions

1. The first thing you need to do if you are going to be using wooden skewers for making the kebabs is to soak them in some water for at least half an hour. This will then help to ensure that they don't burn when placed on the barbecue.

2. Now you need to prepare the pork. To do this you need to place in a bowl the olive oil, garlic, salt and pepper and mix together thoroughly. Once this has been done now you need to put the chunks of pork in to the mixture and toss them around thoroughly so each piece of meat is thoroughly coated. Then you can leave the meat in the refrigerator or to one side for 20 minutes or more. It is best to let the meat stay in the sauce for at least 20 minutes to help it absorb some of it.

3. Whilst the barbecue is heating up now you are ready to start making the kebabs on to each skewer thread pieces of pork with the mushrooms and sage leaves. Ideally you should thread on one piece of meat and then one mushroom and sage leave and continue doing this until all skewers have these ingredients on them.

4. Once the kebabs are ready you should cook them over a high heat on the barbecue for 15 to 20 minutes remembering to turn them often to prevent them from burning. Plus baste them regularly with any of the sauce that remains. As soon as the meat is cooked through then they are ready to serve.

Recipe 2 – Barbecued Pork Steaks

This will really provide you with a very traditional barbecue recipe for that you can enjoy.

Ingredients

4 Pork Blade Steaks that are Between 1 and 1 ¼ Inches Thick
120ml Bottle Barbecue Sauce
80ml Honey
1 Tablespoon Worcestershire Sauce
1 Teaspoon Garlic Salt
½ Teaspoon Dijon Mustard

Instructions

1. In a bowl combine together the barbecue sauce, honey, Worcestershire sauce, garlic salt and mustard. This you will then use to baste the pork steaks as they cook.

2. To cook the pork steaks you need to place them on an oiled grill about 4 inches above the heat source. This will provide them with a medium heat to cook and will also ensure that they cook slowly so more of the moisture is retained.

3. You should cook each steak for around 8 minutes on each side before you then cook them for a further five minutes. But the last five minutes is when the pork should be brushed with the sauce. It is important that you turn the steaks over regularly during this last five minutes to ensure that they are both well coated in the sauce and to help it adhere to the surface of them.

4. Once the steaks are cooked place onto clean plates and serve with a crispy green salad and some nice crusty bread.

Recipe 3 – Barbecued Pork Kebabs

These have a more oriental flavor to them but taste just as wonderful as conventional barbecued pork kebabs do.

Ingredients

2 Kg Boneless Pork Loin Cut Into 1 ½ Inch Cubes
128gram White Sugar
240ml Soy Sauce
1 Onion Diced
5 Garlic Cloves Chopped
1 Teaspoon Ground Black Pepper

Instructions

1. Into a bowl place the sugar, soy sauce, onion, garlic and black pepper and whisk together well. Then to this you add the diced up pork and toss to ensure that all pieces are thoroughly coated in the marinade.

2. Now cover the bowl over and place in the refrigerator for at least 2 hours. However if you really want the meat to taste even much sweeter then allow the pork to remain in the marinade overnight.

3. Whilst you are preparing the kebabs you should get the barbecue ready. Place the grill at a level so that the heat is very hot and make sure that it has been lightly oiled before you place the kebabs on it.

4. On to each wooden skewer, which has been soaking in water for 30 minutes, you thread on some of the pork. Once all the skewers have pork on them they are ready to cook. Ideally you should cook each side of the kebab for between 3 and 5 minutes or until the center of the meat is no longer pink. As soon as the kebabs have cooked you can serve them up to your guests with such accompaniments as coleslaw, rice or potato salad.

Samantha Michaels

Recipe 4 – Honey Mustard Pork Chops

Although these are quite sweet the use of the vinegar, wine and mustard in the marinade helps to counteract some of this.

Ingredients

4 Pork Chops (3/4 Inch Thick Ones Are Best)
90ml Honey
3 Tablespoon Fresh Orange Juice
1 Tablespoon Cider Vinegar
1 Tablespoon White Wine
2 Teaspoon Worcestershire Sauce
2 Teaspoon Onion Powder
½ Teaspoon Dried Tarragon
3 Tablespoon Dijon Mustard

Instructions

1. Into a small bowl place the honey, orange, vinegar, wine, Worcestershire sauce, onion powder, tarragon and mustard and mix together. Now place to one side.

2. Next take the pork chops and make some cuts into the fatty edge of each one. This will then prevent the meat from actually curling whilst it is cooking on the barbecue. However make sure that you don't cut into the fat too far. Once this has been done place in a shallow dish and pour some of the marinade over them before then turning the chops over and pouring the rest of the marinade over them. Cover and place in the refrigerator for at least 2 hours.

3. Whilst the barbecue is heating up remove the chops from the refrigerator to allow them to come up to room temperature. Once the barbecue is hot enough and you have lightly oiled the grill you can place the chops on it. Cook each side of the chop for about 12 to 15 minutes and during this time turning them over at least 3 or 4 times. Each time you turn the chops over remember to brush on any of the marinade that is left over.

Once cooked you can now serve them on a clean plate with say a fresh green salad and a jacket potato.

Recipe 5 – Simple Grilled Pork Chops

The perfect recipe to use when you want to prepare something quick and simple to cook on the barbecue.

Ingredients

4 Pork Rib Chops About 1 Inch Thick
60ml Lemon Juice
3 Tablespoons Soy Sauce
1 Tablespoon Olive Oil
½ Teaspoon Brown Sugar
¼ Teaspoon Freshly Chopped Rosemary
Salt
Freshly Ground Black Pepper
Instructions

1. The first thing you need to do is make the marinade for the chops. To do this in a bowl place the lemon juice, soy sauce, olive oil, brown sugar, rosemary, salt and pepper. Then mix to ensure that they are combined together well.

2. Next you need to place the pork chops in a shallow dish or a resealable plastic bag and then pour over the chops the marinade made just now. Make sure that you toss the pork chops in this mix to ensure that all sides of them are coated in it. Once this has been done either cover the dish over or seal up the bag and place in the refrigerator for 30 minutes.

3. After the 30 minutes has elapsed remove the chops from the refrigerator and leave to one side to come up to room temperature. Also after taking the chops out of the refrigerator now is when you should be heating the barbecue up. As soon as the barbecue is ready you can now start cooking the chops.

4. The grill, which has been lightly oiled, should be placed quite close to the heat source as this will then help to sear the meat and ensure plenty of the meats juices are retained whilst you then cook

them on a medium heat for 6 to 8 minutes. To reduce the heat you simply move the grill up away from the heat source. Also when cooking the chops remember to turn them over regularly to prevent them from burning.

As soon as the chops are cooked you should serve them immediately to your guests on a nice clean plate with say a jacket potato and coleslaw.

Recipe 6 – Basic Barbecued Pork Spare Ribs

No barbecue is complete without people having barbecued pork ribs served to them. If you have never tried cooking such food before this is one of the simplest recipes you can use.

Ingredients

1.36 Kg Pork Spare Ribs
240ml Ready Made Barbecue Sauce

Instructions

1. Take the ribs and place them over a low heat on the barbecue and cook for between 1 and 1 ½ hours. You could of course cut down the cooking time if you wish by initially cooking them in the oven.

2. About 15 minutes before you then remove the pork spare ribs from the barbecue you now start to brush them with the barbecue sauce. It is important that during these last minutes of cooking is that you turn the ribs over and baste them with the sauce regularly. This will then help to ensure that all sides of the ribs get a good coating of the sauce and also will help to prevent the sauce from burning.

3. As soon as the ribs are cooked remove from the barbecue and cut up into portions that people will find easy to eat. Also it is a good idea to serve them with freshly made coleslaw and some crusty bread.

Recipe 7 – Southern Pulled Pork

This is a very traditional recipe enjoyed in the southern parts of the USA. Once cooked traditionally the meat is then served on a bun and some coleslaw. Plus also gets served with lots of hot vinegar sauce.

Ingredients

1.8 to 2.2 Kg Pork Shoulder Roast
2 Tablespoons Paprika
1 Tablespoon Brown Sugar
1 Tablespoon Chilli Powder
1 Tablespoon Ground Cumin
1 Tablespoon White Sugar
1 ½ Teaspoons Ground Black Pepper
2 Teaspoons Salt
1 Teaspoon Ground Red Pepper

Instructions

1. Into a bowl place all the spices to form a dry rub and then press it well into all the pork's surfaces. Whilst you are doing this you should get the barbecue heated up ready for cooking.

2. As soon as the barbecue has heated and you have placed the grill high above the heat source you can now put the pork on to cook. When placed on the grill it will now require between 2.5 and 3 hours to cook. Whilst cooking it is important that you turn the meat regularly to prevent it from burning. Also to make sure that the meat is cooking properly insert a meat thermometer into the centre of it. The right temperature inside the meat, which will ensure it is cooked through, should be 170 degrees Fahrenheit.

3. After the cooking time has elapsed you now need to remove the pork from the barbecue and leave it to rest for around 10 minutes. Then it is ready to be shredded. You do this by using two forks to pull the meat apart and it is this action, which has given this recipe its name. As soon as you have done this place the meat on a clean plate and allow your guests to take a bun and pile it on it before adding some hot sauce if they want.

Recipe 8 – Grilled Pork Tenderloin Satay

If you are looking for a more healthy option to provide your guests with at your next barbecue this is a great recipe to consider trying. However be aware that you shouldn't serve such food to any guests who may have a nut allergy.

Ingredients

450gram Pork Tenderloin
1 Small Chopped Onion
32gram Brown Sugar
60ml Water
3 Tablespoons Reduced Sodium Soy Sauce
2 Tablespoons Reduced Fat Creamy Peanut Butter
4 ½ Teaspoons Canola Oil
2 Garlic Cloves Minced
¼ Teaspoon Ground Ginger

Instructions

1. In a small saucepan put the onion, sugar, water, soy sauce, peanut butter, canola oil, garlic and ginger. Then over a medium heat bring these ingredients to a boil before turning the heat down so that they start simmering and leave uncovered for 10 to 12 minutes or until the sauce has started to thicken. To prevent the sauce from sticking to the base of the saucepan and burning you need to be stirring it regularly.

As soon as the sauce has become thick remove from heat and place about 120ml to one side.

2. Take the pork tenderloin and cut in half width wise before then cutting each half into thin strips than you then thread on to eight wooden or metal skewers. If you are using wooden skewers remember to soak them in water for ½ hour.

3. To cook place them on a lightly oiled grill on the barbecue over a medium to hot heat and cook on each side for 2 to 3 minutes. It is important whilst the kebabs are cooking that you baste them

regularly with the sauce you made earlier. The meat will be cooked when it no longer looks pink.

To serve these kebabs simply place them on a clean plate along with the reserved sauce and allow guests to pick them up and then dip in the sauce.

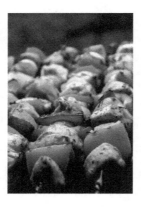

Recipe 9 – Easy Teriyaki Kebabs

These particular pork kebabs can be made in a matter of minutes, as you will be using a ready prepared teriyaki marinade.

Ingredients

900gram Pork Tenderloin - Trimmed And Cut Into 1 Inch Cubes
240ml Ready Prepared Teriyaki Sauce
2 Tablespoons Vegetable Oil
1 20 Ounce Can Pineapple Chunks Drained
500gram Cherry Tomatoes
2 Red or Green Bell Peppers – Cut Into 1 ½ Inch Pieces

Instructions

1. Piece the cubes of pork tenderloin so that the meat can absorb the sauce and oil you are using to marinate them in.

2. To make the marinade simply pour the sauce and oil into a bowl and whisk. However before pouring it over the pork make sure that you keep at least 2 tablespoons to one side in a separate bowl. Once poured over the meat cover and place in a refrigerator and

leave for at least 1 hour. Whilst it is in the fridge make sure that you turn the meat occasionally this will then help to ensure that as much of the teriyaki sauce is absorbed by the meat.

3. After 1 hour remove the meat from the fridge then thread on to skewers. After each piece of meat thread on a piece of pineapple, a tomato and some pepper. Continue doing this until all ingredients have been used up. It is important that whilst you are doing this that the barbecue should be heating up.

4. To cook the kebabs you place them on the lightly oiled grill about 4 or 5 inches above the heat source and cook them on the barbecue for 15 minutes. It is important that when cooking these kebabs you turn them over frequently and brush with the marinade placed to one side earlier.

As soon as the kebabs are cooked served with a noodle or rice salad.

Recipe 10 – Baby Back Barbecued Ribs

You can either start of by cooking these in the oven wrapped in aluminum foil or you can do the same on the barbecue. Then you finish them off by removing the foil and backing on the barbecue.

Ingredients

1.36Kg Baby Back Pork Ribs
1 Tablespoon Brown Sugar
1 Tablespoon Paprika
2 Teaspoons Garlic Powder
1 ½ Teaspoons Ground Black Pepper
120ml Water
350ml Ready Made Barbecue Sauce

Instructions

1. Before wrapping the baby back pork ribs in aluminum foil combine together the sugar, paprika, garlic powder and pepper and rub all other them. Remember to turn them over and coat all sides with this seasoning. Now wrap in the aluminum foil, but leave

one end open, as into this you will then pour the water. Now fold up the open end to seal the meat inside. It is a good idea to leave some room around the meat to allow heat inside to then circulate when the ribs are cooking.

2. When it comes to cooking these on the barbecue you place them on the grill and pull the lid down and leave them there for between 45 minutes and an hour. Once the time has elapsed remove the ribs from the tin foil and then replace them on the grill, which has been lightly oiled.

3. After placing the ribs on the grill you can now start basting them with the barbecue sauce. You should allow them to remain on the grill for a further 10 to 15 minutes. During this final cooking time you should be turning them over every 5 minutes and brushing them with the sauce each time they are turned.

Recipe 11 – Maple Garlic Pork Tenderloin

The adding of garlic to the marinade helps to counteract some of the maple sweetness.

Ingredients

680gram Pork Tenderloin
2 Tablespoons Dijon Mustard
1 Teaspoon Sesame Oil
3 Garlic Cloves Minced
240ml Maple Syrup
Freshly Ground Black Pepper

Instructions

1. In a bowl mix together the maple syrup, mustard, sesame oil, garlic and pepper. Whisk thoroughly to ensure that all these ingredients are combined together well.

2. In a shallow dish place the pork tenderloin and then coat it thoroughly with the marinade that you have just made. Cover the meat over and place in the refrigerator to chill for at least 8 hours. However if you really want the meat to absorb as much of the

flavor of the marinade as possible then it is best to leave it in the refrigerator over night.

3. Whilst the barbecue is heating up remove the pork from the refrigerator so that it can come up to room temperature. Once the barbecue is hot enough remove the meat from the dish and set over to one side. As for any sauce left in the dish pour this into a small saucepan.

4. Now before you place the meat on the grill make sure you have brushed it with some oil first to prevent the meat from sticking to it. Cook the pork on the particular for between 15 and 25 minutes making sure that you baste it regularly with the reserved marinade, which you have heated up in the saucepan for five minutes first. Make sure that you cook the meat on a medium heat otherwise the marinade will burn. Plus of course remember to turn the meat regularly to ensure that it is cooked through evenly.

As soon as the meat is cooked the inside no longer looks pink place to one side for a few minutes before carving and serving to your guests.

Recipe 12 – Maple Glazed Ribs

The sweetness of the maple syrup really does help to bring out the lovely taste of this meat.

Ingredients

1.5kg Baby Back Pork Ribs
180ml Maple Syrup
2 Tablespoons Brown Sugar
2 Tablespoons Ketchup
1 Tablespoon Cider Vinegar
1 Tablespoon Worcestershire Sauce
½ Teaspoon Salt
½ Teaspoon Mustard Powder

Instructions

1. Place the ribs into a large saucepan or pot and cover with water. Then cook on a low heat so the water is simmering for at least an hour or until the meat has become tender. Once the meat is cooked remove the ribs from the water and place them in a shallow dish and set aside whilst you make the marinade.

2. To make the marinade place the maple syrup, sugar, ketchup, vinegar, Worcestershire sauce, salt and mustard into a saucepan. Place on the hob and bring to the ingredients to the boil before then reducing the heat down and cooking for five minutes. Make sure that you stir the sauce frequently then allow to cool slightly before then pouring it over the ribs. Now place the ribs in the dish covered in the sauce in the refrigerator for 2 hours to marinate.

3. You will be cooking the ribs on an indirect heat on the grill so make sure that it is hot enough. Once the barbecue has heated up sufficiently remove the ribs from the marinade and place them on the lightly oiled barbecue grill. Any marinade left over should be put into a saucepan and boiled for a few minutes.

4. The ribs should only need to remain on the barbecue for around 20 minutes. During this time they should be turned frequently and brushed with the cooked marinade often until the ribs have become nicely glazed. Divide up the ribs into manageable portions and serve to your guests.

Recipe 13 –Smoked Pork Spare Ribs

These are slightly sweet but also slightly spicy yet the flavors don't overwhelm the meat, which falls away from the bone very easily when cooked properly.

Ingredients

3Kg Pork Spareribs

Dry Rub Mixture

64gram Brown Sugar
2 Tablespoons Chilli Powder
1 Tablespoon Paprika

Samantha Michaels

1 Tablespoon Freshly Ground Black Pepper
2 Tablespoons Garlic Powder
2 Teaspoons Onion Powder
2 Teaspoons Salt
2 Teaspoons Ground Cumin
1 Teaspoon Ground Cinnamon
1 Teaspoon Cayenne Pepper
1 Teaspoon Jalapeno Seasoning Salt (Optional)

Sauce

240ml Apple Cider
180ml Apple Cider Vinegar
1 Tablespoon Onion Powder
1 Tablespoon Garlic Powder
2 Tablespoons Fresh Lemon Juice
1 Finely Chopped Jalapeno Pepper (Optional)
3 Tablespoons Hot Pepper Sauce
Salt
Freshly Ground Black Pepper

2 Cups Of Soaked Wood Chips

Instructions

1. In a bowl place the brown sugar, chilli powder, paprika, black pepper, garlic powder, onion powder, salt, cumin, cinnamon, jalapeno seasoning and cayenne pepper and mix well together. Then rub all over the spareribs, cover and put in the refrigerator for at least 4 hours to allow the rub to become infused in to the meat. However leaving them overnight would prove even better.

2. Whilst the barbecue is heating up you should now remove the spareribs from the refrigerator and start preparing the sauce. In a bowl you need to place all the ingredients mentioned above and stir together.

3. Once the barbecue is ready before you place the spareribs on the lightly oiled grill you must first place some of the soaked wood chips on to the barbecue itself. Once you have done this you can now place the spareribs on the grill with the bone at the bottom.

Now close the lid and allow the ribs to cook for between 3 ½ to 4 hours. If you need to add more coals then do so.

4. Every hour you will need to baste the ribs with the sauce and also make sure at this time you also add some more of the soaked wood chips to the barbecue. It is important that the temperature within the remains at a constant 225 degrees Fahrenheit to ensure that the pork spareribs cook properly.

You can tell when the ribs are ready to eat as the rub will have help to create a crispy blackened bark on the meat and it pulls away from the bone easily. Simply separate into portions that your guests can enjoy and discard any sauce that may be left over.

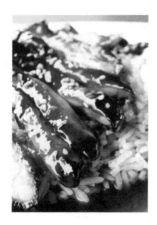

Recipe 14 – Bourbon Pork Ribs

Even though you can cook these ribs in the oven it really is best if you cook them on the barbecue, as this helps to enhance the flavor of the marinade further. Once cooked serve them with a delicious crispy green salad and some garlic cheese potatoes.

Ingredients

1.36Kg Pork Ribs (Country Style Ones If You Can Get Them)
128gram Dark Brown Sugar
240ml Light Soy Sauce
150ml Bourbon
4 Garlic Cloves Minced

Instructions

1. In a food processor or blender place the sugar, soy sauce, garlic and bourbon and turn on until all ingredients are thoroughly combined. Now pour this mixture over the ribs, which have been placed in a shallow dish.

2. Cover the ribs and place them in a refrigerator to marinate for several hours. The longer you leave them in the refrigerator then the more the marinate will infuse into the rib meat.

3. Whilst the barbecue is heating up you should remove the ribs from the refrigerator to allow them to come up to room temperature. But before you place them on the barbecue grate make sure it has been brushed with oil.

4. Once the ribs are on the grate you now need to close the lid and cook them for between 45 minutes and an hour. How long you cook them for will depend on how thick the ribs are. The best way to test if they are ready to eat is to insert a meat thermometer into the thickest part of the rib. If the internal temperature measures 160 degrees Fahrenheit they are ready to serve up on to plates after being separated with the salad and potatoes.

Recipe 15 - Margarita Glazed Pork Chops

This really is a recipe that will excite your taste buds as well as provide you with a food that really does bring out the summer in you.

Ingredients

4 Boneless Pork Loin Chops That Are About 1 Inch Thick
160ml Orange Marmalade
1 Jalapeno Pepper Seeded And Finely Chopped
2 Tablespoons Lime Juice or Tequila
1 Teaspoon Freshly Grated Ginger (If you don't have fresh ginger use ½ teaspoon ground ginger instead)

Instructions

1. In a bowl mix together the marmalade, jalapeno pepper, lime juice or tequila and the ginger. This is what will be used to glaze the pork chops.

2. Before you place the chops on the grill making sure that they cook over a medium heat you trim off the fat.

3. Allow the chops to cook on the barbecue for between 12 and 15 minutes dependent on the thickness of them. The best way of testing to see if they are ready to eat is to insert a skewer into the thickest part and see if the juices from inside that come out run clear. It is also important that you turn the chops over regularly when cooking them.

4. During the last five minutes of the chops cooking this is when the glaze you made earlier must be applied. During this time the chops should only be turned once, but you must apply the glaze often.

5. Once the chops are ready to eat remove from the barbecue and place on clean plates then sprinkle with a little chopped fresh cilantro and some orange and lime wedges.

Chapter 4 - Lamb Recipes

Recipe 1 – Lamb Chops with Curry, Apple and Raisin Sauce

The curry, apple and raisin sauce that you use with this particular recipe helps to enhance the flavor of the lamb further. Plus adds a little bit of spice to the recipe as well.

Ingredients

6 Lamb Chops (Each weighing around 115gram)
Teaspoon Salt to season meat

Sauce

57gram Butter
1 Tablespoon Olive Oil
384gram Chopped Onion
1 Crushed Garlic Clove
2 Tablespoons Curry Powder
1 Tablespoon Ground Coriander
1 Tablespoon Ground Cumin
2 Teaspoons Salt To Season
2 Teaspoons White Pepper To Season
1 Teaspoon Dried Thyme
½ Lemon Seeded and Finely Chopped (Peel As Well)
384gram Apples Peeled, Cored and Chopped
128gram Apple Sauce
85gram Dark Raisins
85gram Golden Raisins
1 Tablespoon Water (If Needed)

Instructions

1. In a saucepan place the butter, olive oil, onions and garlic and cook them over a medium heat until the onions have turned translucent. This should take around 8 minutes to happen. Once the onions are ready you stir in the rest of the ingredients to make the sauce and bring the mixture to the boil.

As soon as the mixture has started to boil you now need to turn the heat down and cover the saucepan and let the mixture simmer for a while. You should check the sauce regularly and stir it also to make sure that it doesn't stick to the saucepan. You will know when it is ready because it will have the consistency of apple sauce and the raisins will start to break apart. Expect this part of the process to take an hour to happen. However if you notice the mixture is becoming thick then stir in the tablespoon of water.

2. Once the sauce is ready you can now go ahead and cook the lamb chops. However before you place on the grill make sure that it has been lightly oiled and that the chops have been seasoned with some salt. Leave them on the grill until the outside has started to turn a golden brown, which should be around 3 to 5 minutes for each side. Of course how long you cook them for will depend on whether you want the meat to be medium rare or medium inside.

To further help test if they are ready insert a meat thermometer into the chop making sure it isn't touching the bone and the internal temperature should have reached 145 degrees Fahrenheit. When the lamb chops are cooked place on clean plates and in a small bowl beside them place the sauce made earlier.

Recipe 2 – Grilled Lamb with Brown Sugar Glaze

Looking for something quick and easy to prepare at a barbecue this summer then this recipe should be tried.

Ingredients

4 Lamb Chops
32gram Brown Sugar
2 Teaspoons Ground Ginger
2 Teaspoons Dried Tarragon
1 Teaspoon Ground Cinnamon
1 Teaspoon Ground Black Pepper
1 Teaspoon Garlic Powder
½ Teaspoon Salt

Instructions

1. In a bowl place the sugar, ginger, cinnamon, tarragon, pepper, garlic powder and salt and mix well together.

2. Now take this seasoning mixture and rub well into the lamb chops on both sides then place on a place and cover. Then place in the refrigerator for an hour.

3. To cook the lamb chops you must remove them from the refrigerator whilst the barbecue is heating up to bring them back up to room temperature and they need to be cooked on a high heat.

4. As usual brush the grill of the barbecue with some oil first before laying the chops on it. Then cook the chops on each side for around 5 minutes or until they are cooked the way you like them. Once they are cooked allow them to rest for a few minutes before serving with a salad and some new potatoes.

Recipe 3 – Mediterranean Lamb Burgers

These burgers really do help to make a barbecue feel even more special. You should serve the burgers in buns with a little salad and feta cheese and also a yoghurt dip.

Ingredients

Burgers

450gram Ground Lamb
225gram Ground Beef
3 Tablespoons Freshly Chopped Mint
1 Teaspoon Freshly Minced Ginger Root
1 Teaspoon Minced Garlic
1 Teaspoon Salt
½ Teaspoon Freshly Ground Black Pepper

Yogurt Sauce

450gram Greek Yogurt
Zest Of ½ Lemon
1 Minced Garlic Clove

½ Teaspoon Salt

Instructions

1. To make the burgers you place the ground lamb and beef in to a bowl with the mint, ginger root, garlic, salt and pepper and stir together until just about combined. Now divide the mixture up into four portions then shape them into four patties. Set them aside. It is best if you cover them up and place in the refrigerator until you are ready to cook them.

2. After making the burgers you are now ready to make the sauce. To do this place the yogurt, lemon zest, garlic and salt into a bowl and mix well. Place the mixture, which you have covered over, into the refrigerator until it is needed.

3. When it comes to cooking the lamb the barbecue should be at a medium heat and will need to be cooked on both sides for between 3 and 4 minutes each. The best way to test to see if they are cooked through is to insert a meat thermometer and see if the temperature inside them has reached 160 degrees Fahrenheit.

4. Once the burgers are ready you need to prepare the buns in which the burgers will be served. The first thing you should do is place a slice of onion and tomato on the grill and cook them until they are lightly charred on each side. Then spread some of the yogurt sauce over the burger or ciabatta roll and then place the burger on top of this. Then place on top of this the onion and tomato slices before some leaves of lettuce. Then top it all off with some slices of feta cheese and the top part of the roll.

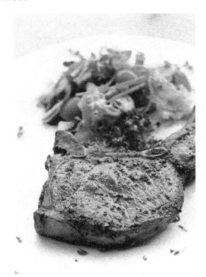

Recipe 4 – Grilled Lamb Chops

Looking for a recipe that will not need much time dedicated to preparing it but will still taste absolutely wonderful after being cooked on the barbecue then you should try this recipe out.

Ingredients

900gram Lamb Chops
60ml Distilled White Vinegar
2 Teaspoons Salt
½ Teaspoon Ground Black Pepper
1 Tablespoon Minced Garlic
1 Thinly Sliced Onion
2 Tablespoons Olive Oil

Instructions

1. In a large resealable bag place the vinegar, salt, pepper, garlic, onion and olive oil and shake well to ensure that all the ingredients have been combined together properly. Then into the bag you place the chops again shake the bag vigorously as this will help to ensure that the chops have been thoroughly coated with the marinate. Once this has been done you place the bag into the refrigerator and leave there for 2 hours.

2. When it comes to cooking the lamb chops you should remove them from the refrigerator whilst the barbecue is heating up. This will ensure that they come up to room temperature ensuring that they then cook properly.

3. When you remove the lamb chops from the marinade to place on the lightly oiled grill if you notice any pieces of onion stuck to them leave them in place. Then grill them until they are cooked to the level of doneness you require. Around 3 minutes for each side should be enough for them to be medium. Once cooked allow to rest for a short while before then serving to your guests.

Recipe 5 – Lamb Kofta Kebabs

These lamb Kofta kebabs don't take very long to prepare or cook and make a wonderful addition to any barbecue.

Ingredients

450gram Ground Lamb Meat
4 Garlic Cloves Minced
1 Teaspoon Salt
3 Tablespoons Grated Onion
3 Tablespoons Freshly Chopped Parsley
1 Tablespoon Ground Coriander
1 Teaspoon Ground Cumin
½ Teaspoon Ground Cinnamon
½ Teaspoon Ground All Spice
¼ Teaspoon Cayenne Pepper
¼ Teaspoon Ground Ginger
¼ Teaspoon Freshly Ground Black Pepper

Instructions

1. With a mortar and pestle ground the garlic into a paste with the salt then the place these ingredients into a bowl with the onion, parsley, coriander, cumin, cinnamon, all spice, cayenne pepper, ginger and black pepper then to this bowl add the ground lamb meat.

Samantha Michaels

2. Once all the above ingredients have been combined together divide it in to 28 small pieces and form them into balls.

3. To make the Kofta kebabs take one of the balls of meat and thread it on to the top of a wooden skewer that has been soaking in water for ½ hour. Then very slowly start to flatten the meat down the skewer until a 2 inch oval is created. Do this with all 28 balls of meat and then place them on a clean plate, cover and put in to the refrigerator for between 30 minutes and 12 hours.

4. To cook the Lamb Kofta Kebabs you need to ensure that the temperature of the barbecue is of a medium heat and the grill has been lightly oiled. Once the barbecue has reached the right temperature place the kebabs on the grill and cook for around 6 minutes, making sure that you turn them over regularly.

Recipe 6 – Barbecued Asian Butterflied Leg of Lamb

As this recipe does take quite a bit of time to prepare this is the kind of meal you should be serving at a barbecue for a special occasion such as a wedding anniversary celebration.

Ingredients

2.26Kg Boneless Butterflied Leg Of Lamb (Ask your butcher to prepare the meat for you)
75ml Hoisin Sauce
6 Tablespoons Rice Vinegar
64gram Minced Green Onions
50ml Mushroom Soy Sauce
4 Tablespoons Minced Garlic
2 Tablespoons Honey
½ Teaspoon Sesame Oil
1 Tablespoon Toasted Sesame Seeds
½ Teaspoon Freshly Ground White Pepper
½ Teaspoon Freshly Ground Black Pepper

Instructions

1. Place the hoisin sauce, rice vinegar, green onions, mushroom soy sauce, honey, garlic, sesame oil, sesame seeds, white and black

pepper into a resealable plastic bag and shake vigorously as this will help to ensure that all the ingredients are mixed together properly.

2. Once you have made the marinade now place the leg of lamb into the bag also and seal it and move the bag around to ensure that all the meat is coated in the marinade. After doing this you should place the bag in the refrigerator for at least 8 hours. But it is best to leave it in the bag in the refrigerator overnight.

3. Whilst the barbecue is heating up you should now remove the meat from the refrigerator and leave it in the bag until the barbecue is hot enough to cook the meat on it.

4. Before placing the meat on the grill brush some oil over its surface and then place the lamb on top. Any marinade left over should be discarded.

5. You should be looking to cook each side for of the meat for around 15 minutes or until you feel it done to the way you enjoy eating lamb. If you are unsure if the lamb is ready and you have a meat thermometer then insert this to check the internal temperature. The meat should be ready when the internal temperature has reached 145 degrees Fahrenheit.

6. As soon as the lamb is cooked remove from the heat and place on a clean plate and allow it to rest for 20 minutes, remembering to keep it covered whilst resting. Then slice and serve.

Recipe 7 – Summer Lamb Kebabs

A very unusual recipe but one that really helps to enhance the beautiful flavors of the lamb

Ingredients

2.26Kg Boneless Lamb Shoulder Cut Into 1 Inch Chunks
6 Tablespoons Dijon Mustard
4 Tablespoons White Wine Vinegar
4 Tablespoons Olive Oil
½ Teaspoon Salt

½ Teaspoon Freshly Ground Black Pepper
½ Teaspoon Freshly Chopped Rosemary
½ Teaspoon Dried Crumbled Sage
4 Garlic Cloves Chopped
4 Green Bell Peppers Cut Into Large Chunks
1 Packet Fresh Whole Mushrooms (The Button Type Are Ideal)
1 Can Pineapple Chunks (Juice Drained But Retained)
256gram Cherry Tomatoes
4 Onions Cut Into Quarters
1 Jar Maraschino Cherries (Juice Drained But Retained)
76gram Butter Or Margarine Melted

Instructions

1. In a large bowl put the chunks of lamb ready for the marinade to be added to them.

2. To make the marinade place the mustard, vinegar, olive oil, salt, pepper, sage, rosemary and garlic and mix well together before then pouring over the lamb. Use your hands and mix all these ingredients together to make sure that all parts of the lamb are then coated in the marinade. Once you have done this cover the bowl over and place in the refrigerator overnight.

3. Whilst the barbecue is heating up you can now start to make the kebabs. If you are using wooden skewers make sure that they have been soaking in some water for at least 30 minutes. To make each kebab thread on pieces of meat along with some of the mushrooms, tomatoes, pineapple and cherries and then place on the lightly oiled barbecue grill to cook. Each kebab should remain on the barbecue for around 12 minutes and you should be turning them over frequently to prevent them from burning.

4. It is important that whilst cooking the kebabs that you baste them with a sauce made from the melted butter, pineapple and cherry juice. This will help to enhance the flavor not only of the lamb but the other ingredients on the kebabs.

Recipe 8 – Herb Marinated Lamb Chops

Although this recipe requires the lamb chops to remain in the marinade for 8 hours or more it helps to make the meat much more tender. Plus helps the marinade being absorbed by the meat and so helps to bring out more of its flavor.

Ingredients

4 Lamb Loin Chops Bone In (1 Inch Thick)
60ml Dry Red Wine
2 Tablespoons Sodium Reduced Soy Sauce
1 ½ Teaspoons Fresh Minced Basil
½ Teaspoon Freshly Ground Pepper
1 Minced Garlic Clove

Instructions

1. In a large plastic resealable bag mix together the wine, soy sauce, basil, mint, garlic and pepper. Once thoroughly mixed together pop the chops into the bag and shake the bag so that all parts of the chops are coated in the refrigerator. Now seal the back up and place in the refrigerator for at least 8 hours. However if you have enough time available leave them in the refrigerator overnight.

2. Whilst the barbecue is heating up remove the lamb chops from the refrigerator and from the bag. Any marinade left in the bag should be discarded.

3. Once the barbecue is at the right temperature you need to be cooking the lamb chops over a medium heat with the cover up. To cook the chops on a medium heat the grill, which has been lightly oiled, should sit about 4 to 6 inches above the heat source. Now cook each side of the chop for between 5 and 7 minutes or until the meat has reached the way you like lamb to be cooked.

When the lamb chops are cooked remove from heat and let them rest for a short while before serving. A good accompaniment to serve with this particular recipe would be some couscous.

Samantha Michaels

Recipe 9 – Grilled Indian Style Lamb Chops

These particular lamb chops after being removed from the marinade will need to be cooked hot and fast. A good accompaniment to serve with this particular dish would be some rice or some grilled vegetables.

Ingredients

12 Lamb Rib Chops
60ml Water
3 Tablespoons Vegetable Oil
2 Tablespoons Curry Powder
1 Tablespoon White Vinegar
2 Teaspoons Onion Powder
1 Teaspoon Garlic Powder
1 Teaspoon Garam Masala
¼ Teaspoon Salt

Instructions

1. Place the 12 lamb rib chops into a shallow dish. Now in a bowl mix together the oil, curry powder, white vinegar, onion and garlic powder, the garam masala and salt and then pour this over the lamb chops. It is a good to pour ½ the marinade over first then turn the chops over and pour the rest of the marinade over them.

2. You now need to place the dish, which you have covered over, in the refrigerator for 1 to 3 hours. Remove them from the refrigerator at least 15 minutes before required in order to bring the meat back up to room temperature.

3. Whilst waiting for the chops to comeback up to room temperature now is when you should light the barbecue so it will be hot enough for you to then cook the lamb rib chops on it very quickly. In fact you need to cook the lamb chops on the barbecue on a medium heat so the grill should sit around 4 to 6 inches above the heat source.

4. When it comes to cooking the lamb chops they should be cooked on each side for 4 minutes. However before you place them on the

grill make sure that you have oiled it well. Once the chops are cooked they can be served immediately with either some chutney or a yogurt sauce.

Recipe 10 – Moroccan Leg of Lamb

Not only is this an exotic way to serve a leg of lamb to your guests but also a very flavorsome way.

Ingredients

1.36 to 1.81Kg Boneless Leg of Lamb
43gram Freshly Chopped Cilantro
32gram Freshly Chopped Mint
60ml Olive Oil
2 Minced Garlic Cloves
2 Teaspoons Ground Coriander
1 Teaspoon Freshly Grated Ginger
1 Teaspoon Salt
½ Teaspoon Chilli Powder

Instructions

1. In a small mix together the oil, cilantro, mint, garlic, coriander, ginger, salt and chilli powder.

2. Place the boneless leg of lamb into a shallow dish and then pour over the marinade you have just made. Cover the dish with some aluminum foil and place in the refrigerator for it to then marinate for between 2 and 4 hours.

3. When the time comes to remove the lamb from the refrigerator you should now start heating up the barbecue. Make sure that it is heated up to a temperature that allows you to cook the lamb on a medium to low heat.

4. As soon as the barbecue is ready place the leg of lamb on to the grill, which has been oiled before, and cook directly above the heat source for 20 to 30 minutes or until it has cooked to the way you like it. Once the lamb has cooked remove from the barbecue and place on a clean plate to rest for 10 minutes before you then carve

and serve it. A nice accompaniment to this particular dish would be a fresh green bean salad and some couscous or rice.

Recipe 11 – South African Lamb and Apricot Sosaties (Kebabs)

This is a very traditional style of South African barbecue (braai) dish and if you want you can replace the lamb with beef or venison.

Ingredients

200gram Diced Lamb
225gram Low Fat Natural Yogurt
350gram Dried Apricots
1 Dessertspoon Curry Powder
1 Tablespoon Caster Sugar
1 Tablespoon Vegetable Oil
1 Large Onion

Instructions

1. In a bowl combine together the yogurt; curry powder, sugar and oil to make a sauce. Add as much salt and pepper to this to season.

2. Take the onion and cut this in 1 ¼ inch pieces which you will then thread on to the skewers alternately with the diced lamb and the dried apricots. If you are going to be using wooden skewers then make sure that you soak them in some water for around 30 minutes before you make the Sosaties.

3. Once you have threaded all the lamb, apricot and onions on to the skewers place them in a large plastic resealable bag or a container then pour the sauce you made previously all over them. If you need to do turn the kebabs over to ensure that they are well coated with the sauce that you are now going to marinate them in. You can either leave them to marinate in the sauce for 8 hours. However if you want the Sosaties to become infused with lots of the marinates flavor it is best to leave them in it in a refrigerator over night.

4. When it comes to cooking the Sosaties preheat the barbecue to a medium heat and just before you lay the Sosaties on the grill brush it with some oil. Cook the Sosaties on the grill for 8 to 10 minutes on each side. Then remove from the heat and serve immediately to your guests.

Recipe 12 – Greek Lamb Chops

Not only are these lamb chops packed with loads of flavor if you leave them in the marinade for sometime they come out tasting extremely tender.

Ingredients

8 Lamb Chops
120ml Olive Oil
120ml Red Wine Vinegar
32gram Freshly Chopped Mint
3 Cloves Garlic Minced
1 Teaspoon Salt
1 Teaspoon Freshly Ground Black Pepper

Instructions

1. In a bowl combine together the olive oil, red wine vinegar, freshly chopped mint and minced garlic cloves. Now pour this mixture (marinade) into a bag that is resealable and to this add the lamb chops. Move the chops around inside the bag to ensure that they are well coated in the marinade and place in the refrigerator. Leave them there for 2 hours.

2. After removing the lamb chops from the refrigerator you should pre heat the barbecue in readiness for when they will need cooking.

3. Before placing the lamb chops on the grill you should season with a little salt and pepper. Then after making sure that the grill of the barbecue is about 3 inches above the heat source you should oil it lightly before placing the chops on it.

4. You should cook each chop for 5 to 6 minutes on each side. It is a good idea to turn them over regularly to prevent them from burning rather than just charring. Once the cooking time has elapsed remove from heat and place on a clean plate to rest for a few minutes. Then serve them with some pitta bread, yogurt dip and a Greek salad.

Recipe 13 – Grilled Rack of Lamb

The marinade you make for this particular dish helps to give the lamb a much sweeter and tarter flavor helping to enhance the meat even more.

Ingredients

1 Rack Of Lamb
240ml Red Currant Jelly
240ml Dijon Mustard
240ml White Wine (Dry or Medium Would Be Best)
64gram Butter
64gram Minced Shallots
2 Tablespoons Fresh Crushed Rosemary

Instructions

1. In a saucepan place the red currant jelly and mustard and simmer on a low heat for about 5 minutes or until the jelly has melted. Then allow the sauce to cool completely.

2. Cut the rack of lamb into chops and then French cut. If you are not able to do this then get your butcher to do it for you. It is important if you decide to do this yourself that you don't remove any of the fat from the eye of the chop. This fat actually helps to prevent the meat from burning when you place it on the barbecue grill.

3. Once the rack of lamb is ready you now submerge it completely in the sauce you made earlier and leave it in it to marinade overnight. Cover the dish in which the lamb has been placed and put in the refrigerator.

4. When it comes to cooking the lamb it should be done over a medium to high heat and with some hickory coals added to the barbecue beforehand. Also make sure that the grill has been oiled before the lamb is placed on it. Cook on the barbecue for 4 to 5 minutes on each side and basting each side regularly with more of the marinade sauce.

5. Whilst the lamb is resting you can now prepare the garnish to go with them. In a saucepan place the butter and allow it to melt over a low heat then add the minced shallots to it. Allow the shallots to brown before then adding the crushed rosemary and white wine.

As soon as the garnish is ready place the lamb on clean plates and serve with the garnish poured over it and with grilled vegetables and potatoes.

Recipe 14 – Greek Burgers

To further add a real Greek feel to these burgers it is a good idea to add some feta cheese to the top of burgher just before serving.

Ingredients

450gram Ground Lamb
1 Tablespoon Dijon Mustard
1 Tablespoon Fresh Lemon Juice
1 Tablespoon Minced Onion
1 Garlic Clove Minced
½ Teaspoon Crushed Dried Rosemary
½ Teaspoon Salt (To Taste)
¼ Teaspoon Freshly Ground Pepper

To Serve

4 Hamburger Rolls or Pitta Breads
Cucumber Slices
Tomato Slices
Onion Slices

Instructions

1. In a bowl mix together the ground lamb, mustard, lemon juice, onion, garlic, rosemary, salt and pepper. You can of course combine these ingredients by hand otherwise you may want to consider using a food processor.

2. Once all the above ingredients have been combined together you now need to divide into four equal portions and then form patties out of each one. It is important that whilst you are making these Greek burgers that you turn the barbecue on or light the coals so it is at the right temperature for you to then cook the burgers.

3. Before you place the burgers on the grill lightly oil its surface with some olive oil and grill until you notice the burgers are no longer pink in color. On average you should expect it to take around 10 minutes for these burgers to be cooked properly. Remember to turn them over at least once.

4. Just before you take the burgers off the grill place the pitta breads or burger buns on it to become warmed through. Then when they are ready place the burgers on them and top with slices of cucumber, tomato and onion. You may also want to consider adding a light yogurt and mint dressing to them as well.

Recipe 15 – Teriyaki Lamb Kebabs

Most people wouldn't consider using teriyaki sauce on lamb but it does actually compliment the meat very well. These lamb kebabs make a wonderful meal for a warm summer evening when served with some rice.

Ingredients

680gram Boneless Lamb Cut Into 1 Inch Cubes
3 Bell Peppers (1 Red, 1 Yellow and 1 Green) Deseeded And Cut Into 1 Inch Pieces
2 Medium Red Onions Cut Into 1 Inch Pieces
8 Cap Mushrooms
1 Pineapple Cut Into 1 Inch Pieces

Marinade

60ml Red Wine
2 Tablespoons Olive Oil
2 Tablespoons Teriyaki Sauce
4 Cloves of Garlic Minced
Grated Rind Of 1 Lemon
1 Teaspoon Freshly Ground Black Pepper
½ Teaspoon Ground Ginger (Fresh If Possible)

Instructions

1. In a bowl mix together all the marinade ingredients then place to one side.

2. Now on to skewers thread pieces of the lamb, peppers, onions, mushrooms and pineapple. Alternate between each item and if you are using wooden skewers then make sure that they have been soaked in some water for at least 30 minutes before you start making the kebabs.

3. As you make each kebab place them in a shallow dish and when all have been made you can now pour over the marinade. Pour over the marinade a little at the time and turn the kebabs over to ensure that every part of them is coated in the marinade. Now cover and place in the refrigerator for at least 8 hours. Whilst they are in the refrigerator make sure that you turn them over occasionally to ensure that all sides of the kebabs remain coated in the marinade.

4. After removing the lamb kebabs from the refrigerator you should start your barbecue up this will then allow time for the kebabs to reach room temperature and will help to make cooking them much easier. You should cook them over a medium heat so place the grill about 6 inches above the heat source.

5. Prior to placing the kebabs on the grill apply a little olive to prevent the kebabs from sticking to it. Then brush with some of the left over marinade and cook for between 12 and 15 minutes. Whilst they are cooking make sure that you turn them over at least 3 times to ensure that they cooked evenly through. Once they are cooked serve immediately to your guests.

Samantha Michaels

MORE 70 BEST EVER RECIPES EBOOKS REVEALED AT MY AUTHOR PAGE:-

CLICK HERE TO ACCESS THEM NOW

CPSIA information can be obtained
at www.ICGtesting.com
Printed in the USA
LVHW061356090619
620638LV00007B/459/P